TO OUR HEALTH

USING THE INNER ART OF DOWSING

IN THE SEARCH FOR

HEALTH-HAPPINESS-HARMONY

IN

BODY-MIND-SPIRIT

Written and Compiled with Love
by
Anneliese Gabriel Hagemann
and
Doris Katharine Hagemann

D1568789

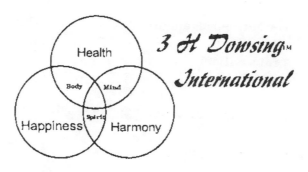

3 H Dowsing International

3H Dowsing International is a trademark of Anneliese Hagemann.

A loose-leaf workbook **To Our Health: Dowsing for Health-Happiness-Harmony in Body-Mind-Spirit,** was published privately in 1996 by Anneliese Gabriel Hagemann and Doris Katharine Hagemann.

It was revised in 1997 and again in 1999, and published with the title **To Our Health: Using the Inner Art of Dowsing in the Search for Health-Happiness-Harmony in Body-Mind-Spirit.**

All rights reserved.
© Copyright 1996, 1997, 1999.
Copyright is owned by the authors: **3H Dowsing International**
                                    Anneliese Gabriel Hagemann
                                    Doris Katharine Hagemann

Author's address: 3H Dowsing International
                             Anneliese Gabriel Hagemann
                             #W10160, County Road C
                             Wautoma, WI 54982 U.S.A.

Telephone contacts
for Anneliese: Tel.   1-920-787-4747 Wautoma, WI (April through December)
                             FAX   1-920-787-2006
                             Tel.   1-602-986-6720 Mesa, AZ (January through March)

E-mail addresses
for Anneliese:

                             **Email Address: ilovedowsing@hotmail.com
                                        anneliese@3hdowsing.com
E-mail addresses   Web Site Address: www.3hdowsing.com**
for Doris:

Web page:

This Workbook may be purchased and used for educational purposes.
The charts in this Workbook may be reproduced with the permission of the authors.
For information write to Anneliese G. Hagemann at the address listed above or go to the Web page.

Cover designed by Doris Katharine Hagemann
Edited by Katheryn J. Wicker
Published by 3H Dowsing International
Printed in the USA by Palmer Publications, Inc. 318 North Main St., Amherst WI 54406
ISBN   0-9656653-0-5
Library of Congress Catalog Card Number   97-090063

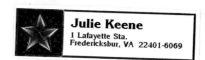
TABLE OF CONTENTS

PREFACE

This Workbook has come together after more than a decade of searching for answers, options, and alternatives. Throughout these years, though both Anneliese and Doris have taken different routes and paths, they have come up with many similar answers.

Anneliese, for the longest time, was ill and could not find answers in conventional medicine. Through her introduction to **holistic** and **alternative medicine**, she began to find that there were many answers to problems. Her search encompassed the use of vitamins, minerals, herbs, chiropractors, changing attitudes, and so forth. She was greatly opened to alternatives and thoughts while nursing her father as he died of pancreatic cancer. Her search is not yet complete, for there is always something new to be found.

Doris has spent years exploring religions, belief systems, cultures, herbs, incense, aromatherapy, music, color, art, alternative lifestyles, and so forth. As with Anneliese, her search is never-ending.

This Workbook Can Benefit from Your Perspective

Anneliese and Doris have developed this Workbook for searching out solutions to problems and issues in one's life. The Workbook unifies many ideas and inputs from a great variety of people, places, resources, ideas, and insights. We've left room to expand and modify the Workbook.

This Workbook is not comprehensive–you may add to or modify what we have put together. We are all unique individuals, each with our own perspective and understanding of the universal God, or whatever one chooses to call the higher powers. Differences in views and approaches need not invalidate other approaches or beliefs. Possibilities of healing and understanding are as infinite as the universe. Each person eventually develops their own approach or insights to what they encounter.

If your have ideas, insights or points to add to this Workbook, please contact the authors. We appreciate any input that you would like to share with us.

Dedications and Acknowledgements

This book is dedicated to my friend, Maxine Jannette, who taught me how to dowse; to my mother and father, for giving me strength through adversity, and whose illnesses opened me up to God; to my daughter Doris for her dedication (without her this Workbook would have been impossible); to my husband Rolf (Rudolf) who allowed me to be me and has given me endless support throughout my journey; to my family (daughter Susan, son-in-law Kevin, grandson Benjamin; Doris's children—Jacob, Pepin, Julia); and friends who let me practice on them. And above all, thanks to God, for all experiences, both pleasant and painful, which have helped me grow and develop continuously.

The editor for the 1999 edition, Katheryn Wicker, helped, revised, and retyped this Workbook. Thank you for your tremendous effort so others can understand and use this book more easily. Katheryn called me during her quest for answers about health concerns and then learned to dowse to strengthen her intuition.

It is impossible to note all the sources of ideas, impressions, information and inspiration that have helped us put this Workbook together. We would like to offer a heartfelt thanks to all of the sources and to God (Great Spirit) for whom we are but an instrument.

Thanks to all. Bless Love. Anneliese and Doris

INTRODUCTION

Healing Your Body, Mind, and Spirit

People are structural, electrical, chemical, magnetic, spiritual, and psychological beings. There must be a **balance** among all of these features. <u>**Balancing**</u> is the key word of nature and health. Once awareness of **balance** is gained, and effort is made to heal oneself, the natural healing process takes over.

If there is **no balance**, dis-ease or disharmony may result. Dis-ease does not imply there is, as of yet, an organic malfunction. Rather, it implies that some part of a person is not at ease.

Self-healing, as discussed by Edgar Cayce, implies that."...**all power, all healing, all help** must come from **within**." Edgar Cayce also stated "Why consult a physician when the physician needed most is **within**."

Body, mind, and spirit must be seen as unified. They are all interconnected and interactive, each affecting and affected by the other. A person needs to be aware of this interconnectedness. Without this awareness, one can never truly understand or get to the heart of an issue or problem.

(See 1 Corinthians 12:1-26.)

The goal of this Workbook is to help you find your own methods to achieve personal **Health-Happiness-Harmony** in **Body-Mind-Spirit**. The 1947 World Health Organization gave this definition of Health: "Health is a state of complete physical, mental, and social well-being, and not merely the absence of disease and infirmity."

Remember, you are the architect of your life!

> The authors of this Workbook **warn** you that this Workbook is not to be used to diagnose, treat, or cure any rational form of disease or illness. According to some laws only your medical doctor has this right. If you have an "illness", a "disease," or are seriously injured, you should seek competent professional aid or advice.

Dowsing for Your Health, Happiness, and Harmony

Throughout this Workbook, **tables and charts** help you find where an **Imbalance** or **Issue** lies, rests, or is located. To specifically identify the problem, the technique the authors use is **dowsing.**

Society has taken away our beliefs in our ability to tune into ourselves for answers to our issues and problems. More often than not, you are sent to a doctor or psychiatrist to work on these problems, when in reality, you, or a good friend, can be the vehicle that helps you heal. By using dowsing, many of us may find the *missing link* to our Higher Self.

Dowsing is an ancient art, known of and used by humanity even before Biblical times. Note is made of Moses and his brother-in-law Aaron using dowsing (a rod) in the Old Testament (Exodus 17: 5-6; Numbers 20: 8-11). Water witches or dowsers have existed for thousands upon thousands of years. Dowsing was highly regarded and important in many villages. Much of the validity and usefulness of dowsing was obscured as churches throughout Europe began to view it as evil and a witch's tool. It is only in this more open-minded and forward-moving century that dowsing has again come into strong use.

As noted above, dowsing has been mainly used by people for finding water. Dowsing's usefulness extends far beyond that, however. Many people have written a variety of books on applying dowsing throughout all areas of life. (See *Reference* section at the end of this Workbook.)

In this Workbook we focus on applying dowsing in your search for **Health-Happiness-Harmony.**

When dowsing, many feel they are tuning in to their **subconscious mind**—a type of sending/receiving station, which is a tie between the universe and one's physical, mental, and psychic self, as well as the past, present, and future.

The French Philosopher Theodore Simon Jouffroy said, "The Subconscious mind will not take the trouble to work for those who do not believe in it."

Albert Einstein said, "**I know very well that many scientists consider dowsing as a type of ancient superstition. According to my conviction this is, however, unjustified. The dowsing rod is a simple instrument which shows the reaction of the human nervous system to certain factors which are unknown to us at this time.**"

Kinds of Dowsing Tools

There are many different types of dowsing tools that a person may use: dowsing rods (a metal rod bent into an L-shape, its handle covered by metal tubes); forked tree branches; coat hangers; radio antennas; and so forth.

For the purpose of this Workbook, we have chosen what we feel to be the most precise method—**the pendulum**. You do not need a specially made pendulum. It can be a string tied to one of your rings, a bead or needle; a necklace with a flexible chain; or, if you desire, a pendulum purchased from a hardware store or New Age shop. Use whatever you personally prefer.

Of course, there are other methods to use when working with this material. **Kinesiology** and **muscle testing** might be alternative approaches if you feel more comfortable with these. If you feel this is your approach, please consult the texts listed in the *Reference* section at the back of this Workbook.

Don't forget that your personal **intuitions, gut-feelings, and sensing** may prove to be worthwhile tools to consult. The longer you work with this material, the more in tune and in touch you become with your **Inner Self**, and the better you understand yourself and others. You might develop the ability to dowse without using any tool other than your self and your intuition. This might include head, hand, or finger movement, or an inner voice.

Be Open Minded and Aware of Your Motives

The main point is to be open-minded. As you learn to dowse, you may come up with different types of issues or problems than another person. Please understand that there are many perspectives and approaches. Picture a mountain. It may be viewed from the North, South, East, West, above, below, or from within. Each view looks different, and yet each viewer looks at the same mountain.

When dowsing, another point to remember is that **thoughts and emotions** may affect the results you receive. Often the **mind** or **ego** is a filter through which one sees or perceives. This may color or alter your perceptions. Therefore, you need to have a **neutral attitude** when asking the pendulum a question. When dowsing, focus on being emotionally calm. You might also ask the person you are working with to keep a quiet, neutral attitude.

The dowser's intent should be to resolve an issue for the **Highest Good** of the person and other beings involved. Dowsing should be used ethically. That is, it should be used in service, harmlessness, and harmony. Do not use dowsing for your own gain.

Again we stress **inner calm**, **being centered**, and having **no ulterior motives** when working with the material and/or a person.

Issues Can Manifest in Many Locations and Levels

One's self is similar to an onion: You peel off one layer and another layer lies beneath. There may be many layers that need to be dealt with, and it may take more than one session to thoroughly balance.

There are many levels where problems may manifest. For example, emotional problems and distress may not only result from emotional or mental upset. Emotional problems may also result from poor diet, allergies, or other environmental factors. Physical problems need not be caused only by physical things. Physical problems may result from emotional or spiritual stresses.

Also there can be more than one issue involved in an area.

Issues, problems, and stress usually manifest themselves into one or more of these:

• Physical or bodily pains or malfunctions
• Emotional or mental upsets (anger, depression, resentment, anxiety, and so forth)
• Spiritual emptiness or confusion

Issues may also manifest at the auric, etheric, astral, or other non-physical levels, which at present a majority of persons in our society do not understand or recognize.

These problems or issues may be limited to one, two or all areas of existence.

Examples above are possible results of issues; however, they may manifest differently for each person.

> On the following pages, the lists, charts, and diagrams help you in your search for balance and well-being. As you browse and dowse through these lists, graphs, and charts, keep an open mind and heart to your healing process.

GETTING STARTED

This section tells you how to use the Workbook and gives guidelines for dowsing.

How to Use This Workbook

Use exercises and pages in this Workbook in the following sequence:

Page	Title of the page and What to Do
7	*Guidelines for Dowsing*
7	*Ask for Permission and Guidance.* Do this at the beginning of all dowsing sessions.
8	*Balance Your Energy.* Also do this at the beginning of all dowsing sessions.
8	*Phrase the Question.* Follow these pointers when you dowse for an answer to a specific question.
9	*Use the Practice Chart to Get Your Dowsing Signals.* Do this to learn your pendulum's dowsing signals.
13	Using the **Out of Balance Checklist**
	Follow steps 1 through 13 when you want a thorough summary of problems or issues and how to resolve them. The *Out of Balance Checklist* starting on p. 14 guides you through steps 1 through 13 listed below.
14	*Step 1: Prepare to dowse.*
	1.A Get permission and guidance to dowse.
	1.B Find out what healing methods are beneficial. Record the answer near the top of the *Imbalance/Issue Record Sheet* p. 18 and on the *Body Chart* p. 17.
	1.C Ask: How well balanced (from 1 to 100%) is this total being? Record the answer near the top of the *Imbalance/Issue Record Sheet*.
22	*Step 2: Locate the person's physical/nonphysical points affected by issues.*
	To locate areas, use your dowsing tool with the *Body Chart* p. 17 and mark the location on the *Body Chart*.
	Record answers at **step 2** on the *Imbalance/Issue Record Sheet* p. 18.
23	*Step 3: On what level of the person's consciousness does this issue show up?*
	To locate a level or levels on the *Body Chart* p. 17, use your dowsing tool with words listed on p. 23 about levels of consciousness.
	Record answers at **step 3** on the *Imbalance/Issue Record Sheet* p. 18.
23	*Step 4: Find out the amount of stress (Major, Minor, etc.) around the issue.*
	Use your dowsing tool to find out the level of stress. Record the answer (for example, M for Major) for **step 4** on the *Imbalance/Issue Record Sheet* p. 18 and at the top of the *Body Chart* p. 17.

*Using the **Out of Balance Checklist**, continued*

24   *Step 5: Identify the issue or imbalance.*

Use your dowsing tool and the p. 24 summary of Body-Mind-Spirit and Other issues. When you have an indicator from the summary, go to the detail page to get more information.

Record answers at **step 5** on the *Imbalance/Issue Record Sheet* p. 18.

26   *Step 6: How is the issue manifested in/on/around the body?*

Use your dowsing tool and the p. 26 list of body systems.

Record answers at **step 6** on the *Imbalance/Issue Record Sheet* p. 18.

27   *Step 7: Who or what caused this issue?*

Use your dowsing tool and the p. 27 list of persons, beings, and systems.

Record answers at **step 7** on the *Imbalance/Issue Record Sheet* p. 18.

29   *Step 8: When did this issue arise?*

Use your dowsing tool and the p. 29 list of time periods.

Record answers at **step 8** on the *Imbalance/Issue Record Sheet* p. 18.

30   *Step 9: What event or place is the origin of the issue or imbalance?*

Use your dowsing tool and the p. 30 list of locations and events.

Record answers at **step 9** on the *Imbalance/Issue Record Sheet* p. 18.

31   *Step 10: Find clues (words, concepts, mental pictures) to self healing.*

Use your dowsing tool and the supplementary list of clues beginning on p. 31.

Record answers at **step 10** on the *Imbalance/Issue Record Sheet* p. 18.

34   *Step 11: What emotions play a role in resolving this issue?*

Use your dowsing tool and the following lists:

      p. 57 *Emotional Gauge for HHH Dowsing*
      p. 58 *Negative Emotional Influences*
      p. 63 *Positive Words, Statements, Feelings*

Record answers at **step 11** on the *Imbalance/Issue Record Sheet* p. 18.

35   *Step 12: Resolve the issue.*

Use your dowsing tool and the instructions on p. 35 to recommend a method for the client to resolve the issue.

Record answers at **step 12** on the *Imbalance/Issue Record Sheet* p. 18.

37   *Step 13: Check whether the issue is 100% balanced now.*

Use your dowsing tool to find out the % balance for the issue.

If it's not 100% balanced, follow the suggestions on p. 37.

Record answer at **step 13** on the *Imbalance/Issue Record Sheet* p. 18.

37   *End the dowsing session.*

Guidelines for Dowsing

It's important that you conduct each dowsing session with respect and compassion for the client. Also you want yourself and the client to be comfortable and well during the session.

Ask for Permission and Guidance

At the beginning of each dowsing session follow these steps:

1. **Say a prayer of protection such as the following:**
   God Force is in and around me.
   Nothing can hinder or harm me.
   Bless Love, Bless Love, Bless Love.

   See p. 15 for prayers that you can adapt to your style.

2. Earnestly let go of ego's tendency to get involved by repeating the following sentences:

   I let go of ego.
   I embrace God. (Or, *I embrace the Universe.*)
   I channel the truth.

3. **Ask this question: May I? Do I have permission on all levels (listed below) of my consciousness and client's consciousness to dowse now?**

   Conscious
   Subconscious
   Superconscious
   Unconscious
   DUPI
   Soul level

   If you don't have permission, you or your client might need to say a prayer or to speak to the level of consciousness that gives no permission.

4. **Can I? Do I have the ability to successfully dowse in this area?**
   Is this the proper time? (If not, when—later today, tomorrow, and so forth.)

5. **Should I? Is it for the Highest Good of all concerned?**

Balance Your Energy

1. Do the following steps, or ask whether you need to do the following steps. The purpose is to allow your body and the client's body to more easily conduct the energy needed to give accurate dowsing answers.

   a. Drink plenty of water.

   b. Walk outdoors to get fresh air.

   c. Eat some energizing food.

   d. To be grounded, put the tip of the tongue behind the top front teeth.

   e. Breath through your mouth.

2. Ask: Am I in my (First) Name vibration?

3. Ask whether you (or client) need to use the word **"Suppress"** to pull your energy close to you (or client's energy close to self). This is especially useful when you are in a group of people or experiencing interference when hearing a response. See p. 37 for instructions to use the word "Suppress."

4. Clean/clear your pendulum by rubbing it, blowing on it, or talking to it.

Phrase the Question

Ask a question clearly by following these guidelines:

1. Ask only one question at a time.

2. Be precise, specific.

3. Ask the question so that it can be answered with the motion that your dowsing tool signals for a "Yes" or "No."

4. More dowsing questions to consider.
   - Is this advisable?
   - Is this the most beneficial?
   - Is this the truth? Is this the right answer for this issue?
   - Is there something else that needs to be asked or addressed at this time?
   - Do I need to look for a different or more effective way?
   - Is there more than one solution? Should several solutions be used?
   - **For me / for you / for others**: to do   to ask for it   to use it   to wear to drive   to check it out   to go   to answer   to attend to   to honor to respect   to acknowledge   to give   to take   to talk   to be silent to be involved   to join   to make it   to dowse

Using the Practice Chart to Get Your Dowsing Signals

To begin, find your "**Yes**" and "**No**" when you use your pendulum. Just as each person is an individual, so too are the ways in which your **pendulum** reacts to you. For example, Doris's "Yes" is a clockwise spin, and her "No" is a counter-clockwise spin. Anneliese's "Yes" and "No" are the same. For others, "Yes" and "No" might be a vertical and horizontal swing. Your Yes/No may take a totally different form, so please follow instructions listed below to use the *Practice Chart* on p. 11 to find these out before proceeding. It may take some time, but be patient and practice, practice, practice.

There are a variety of dowsing signals a person may receive. Be open to alternative answers that you might receive as you develop your dowsing art.

Steps to Begin Using the Practice Chart

1. Ask for permission and guidance, and balance your energy as described earlier on pp. 7 and 8.

2. Have a mental attitude of open-minded questioning, such as "I wonder what the signals are when I use the *Practice Chart*?"

3. Grasp your pendulum's string or chain at a point three to four inches from the pendulum. You can rest your elbow or wrist on a table.

4. Suspend the pendulum directly above the word **Yes** that's written the *Practice Chart* p. 11. Repeat mentally or aloud the following words:

   "Please give me my **Yes**."
   Then wait several seconds for the pendulum to move or jump.

5. If the pendulum doesn't move, give it a small swing.
   Then ask the question again: "Please give me my **Yes**. Please give me my **Yes**."

   Notice whether the pendulum changes direction when you ask the question.

6. If the pendulum still doesn't move or change directions, follow steps a) and b) below.

   a. Again, follow the steps on p. 7 to ask for permission and guidance and on p. 8 to balance your energy.

   Now, ask your dowsing question again: "Please give me my **Yes**" while you suspend the pendulum above the word **Yes** on the *Practice Chart*.

(continued)

b. If the pendulum doesn't move yet, repeat the following sentences out loud or mentally:
- Is using the pendulum for the Highest Good: for all–for me–for others?
- Now, I ask for my Higher Self to come through.
- Does the answer come from my Higher Self?
- I am not influencing the swing of the pendulum.
- I am now free of the desire to control my pendulum.
- Is my rational self or mind in the way?

Now, ask again "Please give me my **Yes**" while you suspend the pendulum above the word **Yes** on the *Practice Chart*.

When the pendulum starts to swing or jump, it's the motion that the pendulum gives when an answer is Yes.

7. Suspend the pendulum above the word **No** on the *Practice Chart*, then ask "Please give me my **No**." Next, suspend the pendulum above the word **Neutral** on the *Practice Chart*, and ask "Please give me my **Neutral**."

8. At another time, go back to the *Practice Chart* to find out the pendulum motion that responds to these questions:
- Please give me my **Don't Know**.
- Please give me my **Don't Ask this Question**.
- Please give me my **Not at this Time**.

9. If you are comfortable using the pendulum as your dowsing tool, you can skip this step. However, if you want to find out whether another dowsing tool suits you better, follow these steps:

a. Notice the part of the *Practice Chart* that's labeled "Which dowsing tool suits me best?"

b. Hold the pendulum suspended above each word. Then ask the following question: "For my Highest Good, do I need to use XXX" where you say the name of one of the tools. For example, you'd ask, "For my Highest Good, do I need to use intuition?" Then let the pendulum swing.

c. Ask the same question for the other dowsing tools listed in the *Practice Chart*.

10. Mark in this Workbook or on a piece of paper the direction that the pendulum moves for your Yes, No, Neutral and other indicators.

11. As the last step, always say "Thank you" with a sense of gratitude for the guidance.

Practice Chart

Follow steps given on the previous pages about using this *Practice Chart*.

Please give my ---

"Yes"   "No"   "Neutral"

Work on the following signals at home, if you're using this Workbook at a workshop.

"Don't Know"   "Don't Ask This Question"

"Not At This Time"

Which dowsing tool suits me best?

For my Highest Good, do I need to use the following dowsing tool?

Intuition   **Muscle Testing**   **Hands on**

Gut feeling   **Finger Stick**   **Pendulum**

As the last step, always say "Thank you" with a sense of gratitude for the guidance.

USING THE OUT OF BALANCE CHECKLIST

On the following pages are charts and lists that Anneliese and Doris developed over several years. We have designed a step-by-step approach in regards to being a Health-Happiness-Harmony Mediator—an instrument for oneself and others in service of the Highest Good.

How to Apply Dowsing In Your Search for Health-Happiness-Harmony

Remember the following helpful techniques while working through the process.

- Respect privacy and confidentiality.
- Be gentle, clear, and firm.
- Have a positive approach.
- Use the Power of Touch if needed.
- Express your feelings, and help others express theirs.
- Offer reassurance.
- Watch for weariness.
- Respect autonomy.
- Have patience.
- Don't take anger personally.
- Pay attention to life reviews.

Read carefully through and use your dowsing tool to answer questions listed in the *Out of Balance Checklist*. The steps numbered 1 through 13 guide you through the basic procedure to begin your work. As you become familiar with this approach, you may change the procedure to fit your abilities, or you can develop a personal method of your own. Again, we stress that there are many ways to reach a goal.

Use the *Out of Balance Checklist* in conjunction with the *Body Chart* p. 17; the *Imbalance/Issue Record Sheet* p. 18; the list of body systems for *Step 6: How Is the Issue Manifested on/in/around the Body* p. 26; the *Emotional Gauge for HHH Dowsing* p. 57; and lists of issues and their resolutions on that begin on p. 39. This may seem overwhelming at first. Be confident! Practice and perseverance help you work through this material. There is repetition at times because some material fits in several categories. Also, repetition keeps you from constantly jumping back and forth from list to list.

‖ Evolution is the Law of Life. Numbers are the Law of the Universe. Unity is the Law of God. ‖
Pythagoras

‖ As you take your first steps into this material we wish you guidance, protection and love. ‖

Out of Balance Check List
(Steps 1 through 13 with Charts and Lists)
Step 1: Prepare to Dowse.

This is step 1 on the *Imbalance / Issue Record Sheet*.

1.A. Get Permission and Guidance (as described below).

Follow the instructions on p. 7 to ask for permission and guidance to dowse. You might find helpful one or more prayers and thoughts listed on the next two pages.

After you ask for permission and guidance, if your dowsing tool doesn't give a clear indication that you are ready to dowse, balance your energy again as described on p. 8. (Using the word "Suppress," described on p. 37, might be especially helpful.)

If you get a clear indication that you're ready to dowse, go to part 1.B, on this page.

However, if you still don't get a clear indication that you're ready to dowse, you are **not allowed** to work on/work with this person or yourself. **Stop here**. Then ask whether that person or you needs to say a prayer or needs to talk to the blocked level of consciousness to open up for healing. (Levels of consciousness are listed on p. 23.) If it still does not want to give permission, then the level of consciousness is not ready to let go to balance. Tell the person that at this time they are not prepared to let go or to balance. You both need to respect this and not go against the Universal Law.

1.B. Ask: Which of the following healing methods are beneficial?

- **Conventional Methods** (p. 19)
  If this person needs conventional methods, stop here and guide them in the correct direction for their healing.
- **Holistic Methods** (beginning on p. 19)

Record methods that are beneficial, near the top of the *Imbalance / Issue Record Sheet* p. 18 and the *Body Chart* p. 17.

1.C. Ask: How well balanced (from 1 to 100%) is this total being?

This question is about overall % balance for this total being. Ask mentally or aloud questions like the following: Is it less than 50% balanced? Is it 50% or more balanced? Is it 50-60% balanced? Let your dowsing tool respond to each question. Keep asking until your dowsing tool gives a clear indication of the correct percent.

Record the answer at 1.C, near the top of the *Imbalance / Issue Record Sheet* p. 18. (At the end of the dowsing session, following step 13, you'll ask this question again.)

Step 1, continued

List of Possible Prayers and Thoughts to Ask for Permission and Guidance

— ✍ —

God's tool I am. What a great honor. God knows that I can work for him on every earthly corner. I go wherever I am needed, wherever I am sent. My heart is open. My mind is clear. Come, Oh Lord, please take me wherever there is despair.
Amen.

— ✍ —

A person's life is like a piece of paper on which every passerby leaves a mark.

— ✍ —

Please Dear Lord,
Put your pure White Light and Golden Light of Love and Protection in me, around me, and through me, so only positive thoughts enter my mind and positive thoughts come from my mind. Whatever negativity comes from me or toward me, please let it go to you for healing.
Thank you.

— ✍ —

When we seek the best in others, we find the best in ourselves.

— ✍ —

Please Dear Lord,
Put your Pure White Light and Golden Light of Love and Protection around us, through us, and in us. Please help us to find the imbalance on the physical, emotional and spiritual level, so we may move forward on your path of understanding, caring, and loving. Let us do your work on this planet. Your will be done.
Amen.

— ✍ —

Please Dear Lord,
Protect and guide whenever I work with the inner child of my client. Protect this child of yours, so that you and I find the imbalance in and on their body, aura, and energy field.
Please help your child to go home with a better understanding of him- herself and you. Help them to realize that they are miracles, and you only perform miracles. Thy will be done. Please let me be your instrument today.
Thank you.   Amen.

(continued)

Step 1, continued

— ℒ —
Kindness in words, creates confidence.
Kindness in thinking, creates profoundness.
Breathe in Peace, exhale Love.
Kindness in giving, creates Love.

— ℒ —
I do not have to have all the answers. I do not need to see all answers or have all the solutions before I act. I need to take heart and fill myself with thoughts of love, strength, and Highest Vision. I need only to aim for the good of all.

— ℒ —
We can heal everything, but we cannot heal everybody. Only God decides if it is the destiny of this particular person to suffer and to be afflicted or if the troubles are meant to be taken away. If it is allowed to be taken away, help is given from God through the facilitator's (or teacher's) hands.

— ℒ —
God Force is within me and surrounds me. Nothing can hinder or harm me.

Body Chart

① Name _____

Birth date _____

Goals to work on if no issues show up _____

How many issues on the same spot? _____

② Conventional or holistic healing method (pp. 19-21)

_____

(If not enough room, record on a separate piece of paper.)

③ Steps 2, 3, 4 (pp. 22, 23) on the *Imbalance / Issue Record Sheet:* Most important issue; aura layer; level of consciousness; amount of stress (Major, Major/Minor, etc.)

Major: _____

Major/Minor: _____

Minor: _____

Minor/Minor: _____

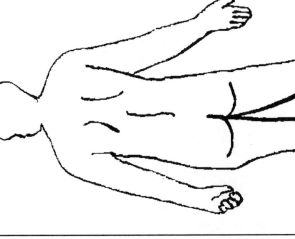

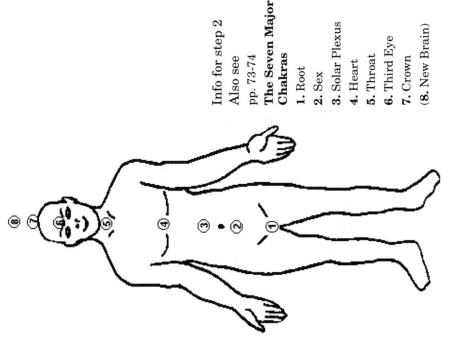

Info for step 2
Also see
pp. 73-74

The Seven Major Chakras

1. Root
2. Sex
3. Solar Plexus
4. Heart
5. Throat
6. Third Eye
7. Crown
(8. New Brain)

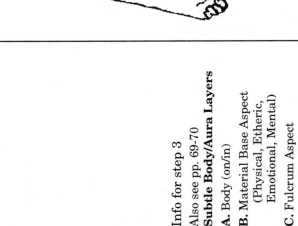

Info for step 3
Also see pp. 69-70

Subtle Body/Aura Layers

A. Body (on/in)
B. Material Base Aspect
 (Physical, Etheric,
 Emotional, Mental)
C. Fulcrum Aspect
D. Individual Soul Aspect
 (Etheric template,
 Celestial; Ketheric, Auric)
E. God Force Aspect
 (1st, 2nd Cosmic Bodies,
 God/Tao Body)
F. Soul-Higher Soul Self

• See step 2 page 22 for instructions to fill in this *Body Chart.*
• Transfer information from this page to column for step 2 on the *Imbalance / Issue Record Sheet* on page 18.

Imbalance/Issue Record Sheet

Name *Anneliese Gabriel Hagemann*   Birth date *9-11-36*   Address *W10160, County Rd C, Wautoma WI*   Phone *920-787-4747* .

☐ Step #1.A   #1.B What Method(s) are beneficial?   #1.C Overall % balance. Before session: _____
(p. 14)   (p. 14)   (p. 14)   After session: _____

Step 2 p. 22	Step 3 p. 23 Level: c sb sp unc du soul	Step 4 p. 23 Stress M, M/m, m, m/m	Step 5 p. 24 Ident. b, m, s, b/m/s	Step 6 p. 26 Manifestation	Step 7 p. 27 Who is involved?	Step 8 p. 29 Time	Step 9 p. 30 Origin	Step 10 p. 31 Clues	Step 11 p. 34 Emotional Gauge for HHH Dowsing — Negative pp. 57, 58 / Positive pp. 57, 63	Step 12 pp. 36, 105-114 Resolution	Step 13 p. 37 Always balance 100%
E	sb	M (Major)	M (Mind)	Central Nervous System	Friend Not my issue	About 2 monhs ago	My yard		Frustrated / Need to provide an ear	This is not my issue. I let go of the frustrated Energy which is held on my Subconscious level of my Being manifesting in my Central Nervous System. This energy no longer serves me. I provide an ear to listen to my friend Maxine. Thank You. Bless Love, Bless Love, Bless Love.	100%

for Step 3:   c=conscious, sb=subconscious, sp=super-conscious, unc=unconscious, du=DUPI, soul=soul, ch=chosen, nc=not chosen

for Step 4:   How much stress is involved: M=Major issue, M/m=Major/Minor issue, m=Minor issue, m/m=Minor/Minor issue

for step 5:   b=body, m=mind, s=spirit, b/m/s=body and mind and spirit, o/u=Ot•er or Unknown at this time

To Our Health: Using the Inner Art of Dowsing in the Search for Health-Happiness-Harmony in Body-Mind-Spirit

Conventional and Holistic Healing Methods for Body-Mind-Spirit

Conventional Healing Methods

A.								
	1	Doctor M.D. Specialist Chiropractor Dentist Osteopath Psychiatrist Counselor
	2	Psychologist Psychotherapist School counselor Guidance counselor Neuropath
	3	Surgeon Eye, ear, nose, and throat specialist Optometrist Opthalmologist Urologist
	4	General practitioner Dermatologist Gynecologist Podiatrist Pharmacist Cardiologist
	5	Orthopedic specialist Endocrinologist Immunologist Test at hospital or clinic

Holistic Healing Methods

B.		
	1	Check books on alternative medicine.
	2	The Complete A-Z Guide: 160 Different Alternative Healing Therapies by Hugh Burroughs and Mark Kastner
	3	To Our Health by Doris Hagemann and Anneliese Hagemann
	4	Energy balance: energy hand-touch healing, vibrational word-energy healing
	5	Cleansing Clearing Life pattern changes Forgiveness Blessings Stroking Other methods listed in *Resolutions* at the back of this Workbook.

(tables are continued on the next page)

Disclaimer: Your vibration of your total Being is calling for this healing method, and it is up to you to seek, research, and gather more information. It is your responsibility and choice to heal yourself.

If required, consult a dictionary, thesaurus, or encyclopedia for clues or key words that might assist with or help pinpoint the problem or issue.

Step 1 and **Holistic healing methods**, continued

C.	1	Nutritional counseling Diets: proper food combination, vegan/vegetarian, eat for your blood type, macrobiotic, pyramid, fasting, living totally on light frequencies
	2	1-2-3 or more meals a day Clearing/blessing your food Acid-alkaline balance
	3	Natural herbs Vitamins Minerals Enzymes Amino acids Teas Spices Cell salts
	4	Flower essences Tinctures Aromatherapy oils, perfumes, incense Wheat grass Kelp
	5	Homeopathic formulas Hanna Kroeger's formulas Supplements Edgar Cayce remedies and healing methods: castor oil packs Body detoxification Dry brush massage
	6	To watch or care for: flowers, plants, animals, birds, fish
	7	Crystals: gems, elixirs, rocks
	8	Herbalist Chiropractor Acupuncturist Homeopathic doctor Colon therapy
	9	Rolfing Massage: deep tissue Urine therapy Shiatsu Color therapy
	10	Reiki Body work Touch for Health Candle ear coning Iridology Biomagnetics
	11	Dowsing Radionics Cranial sacral therapy Zone therapy Therapeutic touch
	12	Myofacial release Kinesiology And many more; check table B row 2, above

Psychic Reading

D.	1	Tarot Medicine Cards Other decks of cards Regular card reading Astrology
	2	Symbology Aura reading Aura balancing Metaphysical healing Chakra balance

Relaxation Techniques

E.	1	Deep breathing Biofeedback Sleep Prayer Meditation
	2	Music Travel Kundalini Yoga Writing Singing Diary Journaling
	3	Visualization Hugging Symbols Nature Laughter Other

Water-related Therapies

F.	1	Therapeutic Sauna Hot tub Whirl pool
	2	Baths: mineral/salt, apple cider, baking soda, Epson salts, peroxide, oils
	3	Herbs Bleach Colon therapy Energized water Remedy water Antidote water
	4	Watsu Fountain Aquarium

(continued)

Step 1 and **Holistic healing methods**, continued

Exercise

G.	1	Yoga Walking Dance Trampoline Bicycling Martial arts Swimming
	2	Aerobics Other sports Play Slant board
	3	How to exercise: physically, emotionally, spiritually Too much exercise Not enough exercise

Group Sessions

H.	1	AA All 12-step programs Dependencies groups: drugs, alcohol, smoking, care giver, child abuse, other
	2	Course in Miracles Transcendental Meditation A Buddhist form of meditation Other meditation
	3	Self Realization Vision Quest Religious Science Church or religious organization
	4	20 Steps to Resolution: Working Mothers, Working Fathers Spiritual group work
	5	A R E Search for God Other

Thoughts and Thought Patterns

I.	1	Positive attitude Affirmations: Louise Hay books, other books, videos, audio tapes
	2	Proper thinking Mental imagery
	3	Guided imagery Loving self Rebirthing Subliminal tapes Other

Goal Setting

J.	1	Volunteer work Career counseling Vision and mission work
	2	<u>Finding your Life's Path/Soul Mission</u> by Anneliese Gabriel Hagemann
	3	Decision making (can be negative stressor or positive stressor)

Psychological Technique

K.	1	Hypnosis Gestalt Focusing Dream work Psychodrama
	2	Past-life regression Rebirthing Jungian psychology
	3	**Writing out for letting go** (can be applied to all levels of consciousness and on all levels of your being)

Possible Sources of Materials and Supplies for Holistic Healing Methods

L.	1	Health food store Food cooperative Grocery store
	2	In home Drug store and pharmacy Garden Book via Mail Family Friends
	3	Relatives Neighbors Holistic health clinic Library Other

Step 2: Locate the Person's Physical/Nonphysical Points Affected by Issues.

This is step 2 on the *Imbalance/Issue Record Sheet* p. 18.

Before starting step 2, follow instructions in *Guidelines for Dowsing* p. 7 if you haven't already done that.

Take from the back of this Workbook the *Body Chart* and the *Imbalance/Issue Record Sheet*. Write the client's name on both sheets. If you are dowsing for yourself, do the same.

Now put your thumb on the name to contact the name vibration of client or yourself.

2.A. Locate the most important issue this being wants to let go of at this time. (See instructions below.)

To do step 2.A, write on the *Body Chart* a small dot on the spot (area) on the front body or back body where the most important issue is manifested. Next, understand which issues to work on as follows:

- In a Workshop, you work on the one most important issue that your partner wants to let go of at this time.
- When you work on yourself, ask how many most important issues is this being willing to let go of at this time.

2.B. Locate the spots on the Body Chart where other issues show up. (See instructions below.)

To do step 2.B, use a dowsing method appropriate to you, and use the *Body Chart* as described next. Ask if there are more issues located on the same spot (area). If the answer is Yes, ask how many issues. (There might be just one issue.) Then draw from that spot outward as many lines the being wants to let go of. Dowse to find which line is the number one (most important) issue. The most important issue needs to be let go first, otherwise work is halted.

Next, ask in which layer of the aura does the most important issue show up? The *Body Chart* lists the aura layers with letters A, B, C, D, E, F. The aura layer gives 1) a further clue about the possible cause of an issue and 2) **where the issue actually started**. For descriptions of layers A through F, see *Aura* p. 69.

2.C. Record your answer.

In column 2 of the *Imbalance/Issue Record Sheet*, write the letter for the aura layer where the most important issue shows up. (In the example on p. 18, the person wrote an **E** for the God Force Aspect layer.)

Regarding what to do next: if dowsing for yourself, you can either go to step 3 p. 23 to continue work on the most important issue, or you can dowse further at step 2 to locate more issues. If you're participating in a Workshop, go to step 3.

Step 3: On What Level of the Person's Consciousness Does This Issue Show Up?

This is step 3 on the *Imbalance / Issue Record Sheet* p. 18.

Issues may not be on a person's conscious level—events during childhood or during times of stress may not be consciously remembered or recognized. Sometimes what a person feels about you affects you without you being conscious of it. Also, people often have a Chosen or Not Chosen in regards to an issue being put upon them.

Thoughts have energy. If the client (you or another person) resists on any level of consciousness about healing, the healing process will not move forward.

Dowse for an answer to the following question: On what level of client's consciousness does the issue show up?

Levels of Consciousness

1. **Conscious** (c)	2. **Subconscious** (sb)	3. **Superconscious** (sp)
4. **Unconscious** (unc)	5. **DUPI** (du)	6. **Soul** (soul)
7. **Chosen** (ch)	8. **Not Chosen** (nc)	

For step 3 on the *Imbalance / Issue Record Sheet*, write the abbreviation shown above in parentheses that corresponds to the level of consciousness.

Step 4: Find out the Amount of Stress (Major, Minor, etc.) around the Issue.

This is step 4 on the *Imbalance / Issue Record Sheet* p. 18.

There is more stress and negative energy tied to a Major issue than to a Major/Minor issue. And more energy is tied to a Major/Minor issue than to a Minor one, and so on. The more energy and stress tied to an issue, the more harmful the issue. More often than not, an infinite amount of negative energy is tied to an issue that's extremely stressful.

Dowse for an answer to the following question: How stressful is the issue—is it a Major issue? a Major/minor? and so forth When you get an answer, write the abbreviation, shown in parentheses, under step 4 on the *Imbalance / Issue Record Sheet*.

1. Major Issue (**M**)
2. Major/Minor (**M/m**)
3. Minor (**m**)
4. Minor/Minor (**m/m**)

When the issue is resolved, it is 100% balanced, and only positive energy is tied to it. If the issue isn't completely resolved, negative energy and stress return. At step 13, we'll check the % balance for the issue to find out whether the issue is resolved.

Step 5: Identify the Issue or Imbalance.

This is step 5 on the *Imbalance/Issue Record Sheet* p. 18.

Dowse for an answer to the following question: Is it a Body issue?/ a Mind issue?/ a Spirit issue?/ a Body-Mind-Spirit issue? / an Other issue? Or do you need to get more clues to identify the area of imbalance? Record the answer under step 5 in the *Imbalance/Issue Record Sheet*.

As a guide or suggestion, the **Body, Mind** and other categories below have corresponding pages listed for kinds of imbalance or influence where you may get more clues, more pieces of the puzzle that puts the life back to wholeness. However, please note that an imbalance may lie in any one of the categories. **Unity** is really what we're dealing with. **Unity=Body-Mind-Spirit**, all areas interconnected and interacting, each affecting and affected by others.

Body (1. Accident, 2. Dis-ease, 3. Shock, 4. Trauma, 5. Neglect)–Starts on p. 39

Page	Name of List	Page	Name of List
41	General Symptoms and Causes	54	Physical.
42,43	Food and Other Allergies		Pathological: organic/disease
44	Atmospheric		Overexertion/exhaustion
45	Chemical		Biorhythm balance disruption
48	Cosmic, Celestial, Planet Earth		Yin (male) Yang (female) imbalance in self
49	Electrical, Polar, Gravitational		Electromagnetic, Potassium/Sodium,
50	Environmental		Acid-alkaline Balance
51	Nutritional		Physiological: fatigue, chemical reaction in the blood
			Psychological mental stress (See *Emotional Gauge* p. 57 and *Influences on Mind Issues* p. 56.)

Mind (1. Accident, 2. Dis-ease, 3. Shock, 4. Trauma, 5. Neglect)–Starts on p. 56

Page	Name of List	Page	Name of List
56, 57	Emotional	66	Intellectual or Mental

Spirit (1. Accident, 2. Dis-ease, 3. Shock, 4. Trauma, 5. Neglect)–Starts on p. 68

Page	Name of List	Page	Name of List
69	Layers of the Aura; Subtle Body	77	Karma
73	Meridians, Chakras	79	Possessive Forces, Entities, Attachments, and Afflictions
75	Belief System/Religious	82	Psychic Senses
		83	Tools and Teachers; Guides and Guardians
		84	Soul Levels

Body-Mind-Spirit (1. Accident, 2. Dis-ease, 3. Shock, 4. Trauma, 5. Neglect–p. 86

Page	Name of List	Page	Name of List
87	Educational Issues	94	Sexual Issues
90	Family Issues	95	Social Issues
91	Financial Issues	105	Resolutions. Also discuss ideas for actions or tasks.
93	Relationship Issues		

(continued on next page)

Step 5, continued

Other

- The issue is unknown at this time.
- The issue is not to be discovered, is hidden, is lost, is left behind.
- There is no problem.
- Do you really want to let go? Are you ready to let go on all levels of consciousness (listed on p. 23)?
- The issue involves surrendering.
- The issue involves self-empowerment.
- These entries may be relevant and are often included within one of the lists given on the previous page:
  - Do you want to die? (If Yes, on what level of consciousness? See list on p. 23.)
  - Fear.
  - Self destruction.
  - Suicidal habits.
  - Feel unprotected (by parents, spouse, sibling, workplace).
  - Unseen influences.
  - Unwanted influences.
  - Engaging in sex, smoking, drinking, reckless driving, drugs, etc.–then playing the victim.
  - A pattern that repeats (3 years, 5 years, 7 years, 10 years, etc.). Often these patterns are installed by others or self.

Are there more clues to this issue?

- In this Workbook
- In another book
- Elsewhere

Step 6: How Is the Issue Manifested on/in/around the Body?

This is step 6 on the *Imbalance / Issue Record Sheet* p. 18.

Dowse for an answer to this question: In which body system listed below does the issue manifest? Record the answer on the *Imbalance / Issue Record Sheet*.

1	**Basic Unit**—the Cell System
2	**Central and Peripheral Nervous System**
3	**Sensory Organs** (eyes, ears, nose, mouth, skin)

4	**Glands**
	• internal secretion (Endocrine–ductless)
	  – pineal, pituitary, thymus, thyroid, parathyroid
	  – gonads (male–testes, female–ovaries), adrenal
	  – all secretory types of hormones
	• external secretion (Exocrine–duct)
	  – liver, pancreas, sweat glands, gall bladder
	  – salivary glands

5	**Circulatory System** (heart, vein, artery, capillary, blood)
6	**Digestive System** (mouth–teeth or gums or tongue, esophagus, stomach, duodenum, small intestine, large intestine, rectum)
7	**Reproductive System** • male—penis, prostrate, scrotum, testes, etc. • female—breast, ovary, uterus, cervix, vagina, vulva, fallopian tubes, etc.
8	**Urinary Tract System** (kidney, bladder, urethra)
9	**Structural System** (skeleton, muscle, ligaments, tendons, etc.)
10	**Respiratory System** (nose, throat, trachea, lungs, bronchial tubes, air sacs, etc.)
11	**Immune System** (lymph glands and nodes, tonsils, immune cells, adenoids, white blood cells, etc.)
12	**Chakra/Meridians** (Root chakra to Crown chakra. See list of chakras on p. 74.)
13	**Energy Field** and **Aura** (See *Body Chart* p. 17 and aura description on p. 69.)
14	**Other Body Components**

> For other possibilities check anatomy books, physicians' references, alternative healing approaches, etc.

Step 7: Who or What Caused This Issue?

This is step 7 on the *Imbalance / Issue Record Sheet* p. 18.

Dowse for an answer to the following question: Who or what being caused this issue? Is there another being or system also involved in this issue?

Frequent Answers for Persons, Beings, and Systems

The next table lists answers that often come up in response to the questions:

❑ Male	❑ Self (the	❑ Spirit	❑ Solar	❑ Alive
❑ Female	client)	❑ Thought form	❑ Planetary	❑ Dead
❑ Male and female	❑ Group	❑ Other	❑ USA	
❑ Male and Male	❑ Family	❑ Unknown	❑ World	
❑ Female and female	❑ Friend		❑ Global	

Example Questions

Please understand the use of the word "client" in the example questions below. If you are dowsing for yourself, you are the client. If you are dowsing for another person, that person is the client.

Listed below is a series of example questions. Adapt the questions to your dowsing session, depending on which answers you get and depending on whether your client is a male or female.

7.A. Who is the primary cause of this issue?

A female?	❑ Yes	❑ No
A male?	❑ Yes	❑ No

The answer would be one of these: a female; a male; or a female and a male together.

7.B. Next ask the following questions until you first get a Yes answer:

Is this the client's issue (asking whether the client caused the issue)?
    ❑ Yes   ❑ No

Is this <u>our</u> issue (asking whether the client and another being caused the issue)?
    ❑ Yes   ❑ No

Is this <u>their</u> issue (asking whether a being or beings other than the client caused the issue)?   ❑ Yes   ❑ No

Are there more clues about the beings involved in this issue?

Is the being, involved in this issue, unknown?

7.C. If the answer to 7.A and 7.B says that only the client is involved, write "self" in column 7 of the *Imbalance / Issue Record Sheet*. (Later, for step 12, the client will write a resolution that begins with the words "This is my issue...".)
Now go to step 8.

7.D. If the answer to 7.A or 7.B says that there's more than one being involved and that one of the beings is the client, you can dowse to learn who the other being (or beings) are. Listed below are a few examples.

- If it's a male and female, ask whether the other being is the spouse or partner.
- If it's a family member, ask whether it is (if gender was given in the answer) mother, father, sister, brother, son, daughter, and so forth, or ask by names of family members. Sometimes a dowsing answer will say the other being is a family member, but the other being is not a blood relative. For example, an answer might say a "twin" is involved, and further questioning then reveals it was a close friend who was born the same year.

In column 7 of the *Imbalance / Issue Record Sheet*, write "self" and a write a word or two for the other being that's involved, for example, "and friend Maxine." (Later, for step 12, the client will write a resolution that begins with the words "This is my issue with..." or "This is our issue..."   And the resolution will mention the other being's name or role.)
Now go to step 8.

7.E. If the answer to 7.A or 7.B says that the client did not create the issue, you can dowse to learn if there is another being or beings involved. For example, a person (the client) might take on another being's issue. In column 7 of the *Imbalance / Issue Record Sheet*, write a word or two for the other being that's involved, for example, "friend Maxine." (Later, for step 12, the client will write a resolution that begins with words "This is not my issue." If you learned that another being is involved, the resolution will also mention the other being's name or role.)
Go to step 8.

Step 8: When Did This Issue Arise?

This is step 8 on the *Imbalance/Issue Record Sheet* p. 18.

Identify the time period in which the issue came about, or identify the time of best understanding of the issue's origin, as described below.

First ask: did the issue arise more than a year ago? Next, ask more questions based on the client's answer. See suggested questions listed below.

Did the issue arise more than a year ago?	
If the answer is Yes: Was it more than five years ago? If the answer is Yes, then jump to ten years, and so on. If the number of years in the past is greater than the person's age, ask if it was generations ago; see suggestions below in row 4. If the answer is No, find out which year, between one year and five years ago.	If the answer is No: Go backwards in number of months. Was it less than 11 months? Less than 10 months? If the answer is a time near birth or before birth, see the suggestions below in row 5 for time periods.

Then ask more questions until dowsing says the answer is specific enough. Record the answer under step 8 in the *Imbalance/Issue Record Sheet*.

Suggestions for Time Periods

1	Past	Present	Future		
2	Hour	Day	Week	Month	Year ago	Year to come
3	Past life	Present life	Future life	Parallel life	
4	Generations ago (miasma) or physical lifetimes ago or incarnations ago (how many?)				
5	In between lives	During conception	After conception	Before birth	During birth

Step 9: What Event or Place Is the Origin of the Issue or Imbalance?

This is step 9 on the *Imbalance/Issue Record Sheet* p. 18.

Identify the physical place or event where the issue arose. Dowse for an answer by asking: Is the origin given in row 1? in row 2? in the table below. When you find the row, ask about each item one at a time until you get a Yes answer. If you need more information about the place or event, you can also ask if there's a clue in row 17. Also see *More Clues* at the bottom of the page.

Record the answer under Step 9 on the *Imbalance/Issue Record Sheet*.

Suggestions for Locations and Events

1	Home (yours/others) Bathroom Bedroom Living Room Hallway Kitchen Basement Shower (in the bathroom/physical needs)
2	Office Work place Farm Factory Business Building Utility building
3	Fun places Amusement park Entertainment Bar Vacation
4	TV Radio Movies Telephone Post office
5	Reading material Correspondence (mail) Dream Symbols or logos
6	Government buildings Church School Bank
7	Shop Flea market Restaurant Store
8	Wedding Wedding shower Baby shower
9	Train Automobile Plane Vehicle Boat Truck
10	County Country Town Village City
11	Lake Stream Dam River Ocean
12	Street, alley, highway Land Yard Mountains Desert Jungle Forest
13	Spaceship Other planet Other dimension
14	Hospital Jail Funeral/Funeral home Cemetery
15	Birth/Death (mine/others) Imprinted while in the womb
16	Animals Other
17	Away Over In On Near Far Distance from place where we're dowsing (inches, feet, miles)

More Clues

For additional clues about origin of the issue, see *Food Allergies* pp. 42 and 43; *Atmospheric Causes* p. 44; *Chemical Causes* p. 45; *Cosmic, Celestial, Planet Earth Influences* p. 48; *Environmental Influences* p. 50; *Physical Influences* p. 54; *Social Issues* p. 95; and the *Table of Contents* at the beginning of this Workbook.

Step 10: Find Clues (Words, Concepts, Mental Pictures) to Self Healing.

This is step 10 on the *Imbalance/Issue Record Sheet* p. 18.

When working on oneself or others, certain words or visual pictures might come to mind. It is strongly recommended that you **make a note** of these because they might provide insight into the imbalance or issue. For example, at one time Anneliese was working with a client, and the word "yellow" came to mind. This proved to be the color of the man's first wife's hair, and the clue showed he had an issue with her.

If you get no clues on this page or pages that follow for step 10, you can also look at the following sections of this Workbook:

- *General Symptoms and Their Causes* p. 41
- *Resolutions* p. 105

Column 1	Column 2	Column 3	Column 4
• Activist	• Age difference	• Assume	• Avoidance
• Addiction	• Argument	• Attitude win/lose	
• Being a puppet	• Blamer	• Bondage	• Bully
• Blackmailing	• Blocking		
• Calculator	• Comfort zone	• Compromising	• Conflict
• Clinging vine	• Commander	• Compulsion	• Confrontation
• Collaborate	• Commitment	• Concord	• Consideration
• Collision	• Competitive	• Condemnation	• Crash
• Defender	• Desire	• Dictator	• Disable
• Doubt	• Delusion	• Dis-ease	• Disease
• Drawn back into			
• Effort	• Ego trip	• Embarrassor	• Evidence
• Failing	• Falling	• Fear	• Feeding into
• Gossiping	• Grief	• Guilt	
• Habits	• Helper	• Hiding	
• Imperfection	• Injury	• Insecure	• Irresponsible
• Incorrect	• Injustice	• Involvement	• Isolation

(continued on the next page)

Step 10, continued

Column 1	Column 2	Column 3	Column 4
• Jailer	• Judge		
• Lifetime			
• Manipulator	• Martyr	• Maskwearing	• Misconception
• Nice guy	• Not believing in	• Not belonging	
• Offender	• Old thought forms	• Oppressor	• Other's program
• Over indulging			
• Parent	• Perpetrator	• Power struggle	• Projection
• Past life vows/ involvement	• Phobia	• Power trip	• Prosecutor
• Pattern	• Pity self / others	• Powerless	• Protester
• Perceiver	• Playing games	• Pretender	• Puppet
• Quitter			
• Reaching	• Rebellion	• Residue	• Risk taker
• Reaction	• Rescuer	• Respect	• Role model
• Reason	• Resentment	• Responsibility	
• Sabotage	• Self empowerment	• Shortcoming	• Surrender
• Sacrifice	• Self program	• Show off	• Survivor guilt
• Safety	• Self punisher	• Sufferer / self	• System
• Self destruction	• Separation	• Suicidal	
• Threats (teachers, parents, etc.)			
• Unprotected	• Unwanted		
• Value			

• Victim—I got sick because of some condition, and I played the victim. Here are some example conditions:

Drinking	Drugs	Reckless driving	Sex	Smoking

• Want	• Weakling	Win/lose attitude		

(continued)

To Our Health: Using the Inner Art of Dowsing in the Search for Health-Happiness-Harmony in Body-Mind-Spirit

Step 10, continued

- Is there a lesson to be learned?
- Does this being want to die? (If the answer is yes, on what level of consciousness? See p. 23 for a list of levels of consciousness.)
- Are you called from the other side from someone?
- What is your belief system?
- Is there dislodged memory (Life) from others?
- Are you speaking woundality (past or future negative programming)?
- Are you carrying this as a privilege for the Planet?
- Are you home sick for heaven–family–relationships–etc.
- Is this being ready to heal? and to accept responsibility in this lifetime?
- Ask first if you have permission to dowse for Soul Level, then ask what Soul Level (p. 84) they are on.
- Does the issue involve an affliction: emotional, mental, spiritual, from possessive force, entity, or other attachment?

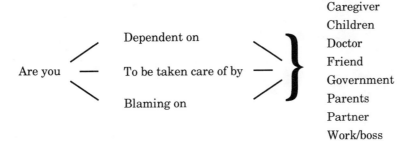

Is this Being choosing to...

Is this Being chosen to...

}

heal self the holistic way?

have the medical field heal them?

ask God/Universe to help?

put their faith in someone else's hands?

Are you —— Dependent on / To be taken care of by / Blaming on —— }

Caregiver
Children
Doctor
Friend
Government
Parents
Partner
Work/boss

Remember, you can also look at the following sections of this Workbook:
- *General Symptoms and Their Causes* p. 41.
- *Resolutions* p. 105

Step 11: What Emotions Play a Role in Resolving this Issue?

This is step 11 on the *Imbalance/Issue Record Sheet* p. 18.

Identifying the emotions around an issue is the most important feature in the balancing or letting go of an issue or imbalance.

To find the most important negative energy that is stored in, on, around the body, refer to the *Negative Energy* listed in the *Emotional Gauge for HHH Dowsing* p. 57. If your dowsing tool doesn't find a word on p. 57, see *Negative Emotional Influences* starting at p. 58. Record the answer under step 11 on the *Imbalance/Issue Record Sheet*.

Now find the most important positive energy stored in, on, around the body by referring to *Positive Energy* listed in the *Emotional Gauge for HHH Dowsing*. If your dowsing tool doesn't find a word on p. 57, see *Positive Words, Statements and Feelings* starting at p. 63. Record the information at step 11 on the *Imbalance/Issue Record Sheet*.

Finally, ask if there are any more clues about emotions that the subconscious wants to give. If you get a "Yes," dowse the *Table of Contents* p. iii for pages that hold more clues. Record the answer or answers under step 11 on the *Imbalance/Issue Record Sheet*.

Step 12: Resolve the Issue.

This is step 12 on the *Imbalance/Issue Record Sheet* p. 18.

Now that you have recorded all the information and clues, review for the client (yourself or another person) what is on the *Imbalance/Issue Record Sheet*.

‖ Don't judge or assume. Accept what Body-Mind-Spirit/our eternal being gives us/you. ‖

Now is the time to balance the issue and transmute or change the negative energy to positive energy.

You or the person you are working with/on needs to take action 1) by writing, 2) by one of the methods listed below under *Ways to Express the Resolution*, or 3) by one of the other methods listed under *Resolutions* p. 105. Merely thinking or speaking is often not enough to complete the letting go. Feel free to intuit or investigate other resources. People with similar imbalances might need totally different approaches to resolve an imbalance.

Ways to Express the Resolution

Is it for the Highest Good of my client (or me, if dowsing for yourself) to do one of these:

1. To write the letting go on paper?
2. To think it out in their mind?
3. To scribble or draw on paper?
4. To dance—sing?
5. To write poetry?
6. To take a walk?
7. To talk to God?
8. That my client and I work through it?
9. To play an instrument?
10. To shout—scream it out?
11. To sing and breathe it out?
12. Putting the hand on where the issue is, to let go?
13. Is the educator to do it for the client?
14. Let it take care of by itself?
15. To accept it as-is?
16. To allow the client to make their own decision?
17. To let go of all the issues at once?
18. To cry—punch it out (for example, punch a pillow)?
19. To do sports, homework, or housework?
20. To work with clay or models?
21. To be outdoors or to work in nature, sand, or soil (for example gardening)?
22. To do hand crafts (for example sewing, woodworking)?
23. To write to the person or people, and
   • to send the written words to the person or people?
   • to not send to the person or people?
24. Food? Laughter? or read books?
25. Does the client have an idea what action to do?

It is best to write out the resolution then take the other appropriate action if an action came up to let go to balance. If the issue does not want to balance, you might want to look for an affirmation or another resolution; see *Resolutions* p. 105 for help. It might take several attempts before the letting go is fully realized. Don't give up too quickly.

(continued)

Step 12, continued

How to State the Resolution

The box below describes using information from the *Imbalance/Issue Record Sheet*.

The first sentence of the resolution

At step 7, you found out whether to state "This is my issue..." or "This is our issue" or "This is not my issue...". Begin your resolution with the phrase that you discovered at step 7.

Mentioning another being that's involved

If it is your issue, and you discovered at step 7 who else was involved, add the following phrase:
"with <name of other being>. I forgive <her/him/them/it>."
This is an example: "This is my issue <u>with</u> Mary. I forgive her."

If it is not your issue, and you discovered a clue about the situation and who caused the issue, write a sentence like this: "I <...do something, at some time...> regarding <name of person or being>." For example, "I send thoughts of kindness to Susan." or "I am assertive with John at work."

The resolution if it is your issue

This is my issue with *name/being*. I forgive *her/him/it/them*. I let go of the (*negative energy word from step 11*) energy, which is held on (*level of consciousness from step 3*) of my Being and is manifested in my (*part of body from step 6*). This energy no longer serves me. I am now feeling (*positive-energy word from step 11*). Bless Love, Bless Love, Bless Love."

The resolution if it is not your issue

This is not my issue. I let go of the (*negative energy word from step 11*) energy, which is held on (*level of consciousness from step 3*) of my Being and is manifested in my (*part of body from step 6*).This energy no longer serves me. I am now feeling (*positive-energy word from step 11*). *Sentence here about the situation and being involved.* Bless Love, Bless Love, Bless Love."

We use Bless Love to fill the void created when we let go negative energy. Your dowsing tool might tell you or client to write Bless Love many times to balance 100%. This is only a recommendation to write a letting go of the issue. You might find different ways to write a resolution that fits the client's needs. Again feel free to do what suits you. For more ideas, go to the *Table of Contents* p. iii, and dowse for a page number to turn to.

Example Resolutions

In the following example resolution, it is the client's issue:

> This is my issue with Mary. I forgive her. I let go of the depressed (*a negative-energy word*) energy which is held on the level of Superconscious of my Being and manifested in my glands. This energy no longer serves me. I am now feeling perfect (*positive-energy word*). Bless Love, Bless Love, Bless Love.

In the following example, it is someone else's issue (not the client's issue), but the client has taken it upon herself and manifested it in her immune system:

> This is not my issue. I let go of the frustrated energy which is held on the Subconscious level of my Being and manifested in my Central Nervous System. This energy no longer serves me. I provide an ear for listening to my friend Maxine.
> Bless Love, Bless Love, Bless Love.

Step 13: Check whether the Issue is 100% Balanced Now.

This is step 13 on the *Imbalance/Issue Record Sheet* p. 18.

Ask to what % the issue or imbalance is resolved. If the issue is not yet balanced 100%, ask the following questions, and use your dowsing tool to get an answer:

- Do you need to find another negative energy to balance?
- Is there another issue or more issues to let go?
- Do you need to find another positive energy to balance the issue?
- Does the client need to write additional "Bless Love" phrases as part of the resolution?

Be sure that the issue/issues are balanced 100%. If not balanced, they grow again.

The client (you or another person) might not feel well after balancing because of toxin or energy shifting into the bloodstream or because of energy blockages that have been freed. The body needs time to adjust. A feeling of tiredness might also be present.

End the Dowsing Session

Check the overall % balance for this total being now to compare with your results at step 1. Record the answer at the top of the *Imbalance/Issue Record Sheet*, at the line marked 1.C, % Balance after. If no other issues remain to resolve at this time, and if the client's energy is in balance, ask for or work toward goal evaluation or goal setting. Here are example questions:

- What do you wish to accomplish or achieve?
- What is holding you back? Is it a past lifetime?
- Is this goal for your Highest Good?
- Do you need to consult the book <u>Your Life's Path/Soul Mission?</u> published by Anneliese Gabriel Hagemann in 1999.

Give thanks for guidance received during this dowsing session.

Special Note: Use Suppress if You're Not Able to Get a Reading

At times, you might not get a reading for the client (yourself or another person). Sometimes the cause of this may be your own (or the other's) high level of energy. Or, you may be too close to a person relationship-wise, and because of your feelings toward the person, the physical nearness of that person may interfere with your receptivity while dowsing—your thoughts and feelings get in the way.

You may need to write the word "**Suppress**" on a piece of paper. If the client is another person, you can place it on the person or on their chart, photo, etc. Or you can hold the piece of paper between your thumb and index finger. This assists in getting through to find the issue or problem. And, if working with another, it suppresses your involvement them.

2

INFLUENCES ON BODY ISSUES

Table of Contents

General Symptoms and Their Causes

Listed next are some general symptoms and categories of influences that can cause symptoms in the body. Also, the causes (influences) of symptoms are listed on pages that follow.

General Symptoms for Body Part or Body Function

Do any words listed below describe symptoms that afflict the body part or function?

Column 1	Column 2	Column 3	Column 4	Column 5
• Congested	• Cold/hot/warm/ normal	• Exhausted	• Frustrated	• Hyperactive
• Hypoactive	• Inflamed	• Irritated	• Malfunctioning	• Needs adjustment
• Overenergized	• Overexerted	• Overextended	• Overworked	• Pressure
• Sprain	• Stagnant	• Strain	• Underenergized	• Underworked
• Unfelt	• Unseen			

Causes of Body Symptoms

Causes of symptoms are listed below and in detail on pages that follow.

Column 1	Column 2	Column 3
• Food and other allergies pp. 42,43	• Atmospheric p. 44	• Chemical p. 45
• Cosmic, Celestial, Planet Earth p. 48	• Electrical p. 49	• Environmental p. 50
• Nutritional p. 51	• Physical p. 54	

Possible Ways that You Assimilate (Take in) the Cause of Symptoms

Column 1	Column 2	Column 3
• You inhale	• You respond to	• You feel
• You put on body	• You follow	• You hear
• You put in your body	• You protect	• You see
• You eat or drink from	• You hide	• You taste
• You store in	• You correspond to	• You smell
• You live in	• You reject	• You underestimate
• You wear close to skin	• You attract	• You deny, dismiss
• You touch	• You collect	• You sense
• You sleep on or near	• You inhibit	• You believe in/ disbelieve
• You travel with	• You inhabit	• You have been sitting too long
• You walk or drive by/on	• You know/ know of	• You need to walk
• You acknowledge	• You sit next to	• You need to work
• You understand		

Symptoms of Food Allergies and Other Allergies

This is a list of symptoms that can manifest in the body because of allergies. (See also other lists on pages that follow.)

Symptoms in the Body

1	Entire system (general symptoms)	Chronic fatigue; weakness after eating; urinary tract (frequency or urgency) hunger or cravings; binge eating; pains and aches in muscles and joints; water retention; swelling of ankles, feet, or hands; lethargy
2	Skin	Eczema; dermatitis; hives; unusual skin pallor; rashes
3	Gastrointestinal tract	Bloating after meals; belching; passing gas; colitis; constipation; diarrhea; nausea; gagging; vomiting; abdominal cramps or pains; stomach still feels full several hours after a meal.
4	Eyes, ears, nose, and throat	Ear ache; fullness in ears; ringing in ears; itching ear; ear draining fluid in middle ear; hearing loss; recurring ear infections; blurry vision; watery eyes; excessive mucus; canker sores; sinusitis; sore throat; chronic cough; roof of mouth itching; hoarseness.
5	Head	Feeling faint or dizzy; headaches; insomnia. Feeling a fullness in the head. Excessive sleepiness or drowsiness soon after eating.
6	Heart and lungs	Increased heart rate; rapid heart rate; palpitations; congestion in the chest; asthma.

Symptoms in the Mind

1	Psychological	Depression; irritability; mental dullness; confusion; anxiety; aggressive behavior; hyperactivity; restlessness; excessive daydreaming; learning disabilities; poor work habits; speech problems; indifference; inability to concentrate.

Foods that Can Cause Allergies

Listed below are general categories of foods. Many people are allergic to or react to one or more of the foods.

1	Amino acids (see p. 53)
2	Antioxidants
3	Birds and their eggs: chicken, duck, goose, turkey, etc.
4	Carbohydrates
5	Dairy products: butter, cheese, cottage cheese
6	Enzymes (see p. 53)
7	Fats
8	Fruits: dried, fresh, juices, etc.
9	Grains: corn, millet, rice, rye, wheat, etc.
10	Liquids: alcohol, beverages, coffee, water, tea, etc.
11	Mammal meat: beef, lamb, pork, etc.
12	Meats of nuts, seeds, etc.
13	Minerals (see p. 53)
14	Natural food supplements
15	Oil: canola, corn, olive
16	Proteins
17	Seafood
18	Snacks of any kind
19	Spices, herbs, condiments, etc.
20	Sweets: honey, raw sugar, white sugar, etc.
21	Vegetables: dried, fresh, juices, soup, etc.
22	Vitamins (see p. 53)

‖ Please note that the preceding list is not a comprehensive list of all food allergens. ‖

Atmospheric Causes of Body Issues and Their Resolutions

Disturbances in or disturbances transmitted by atmosphere can result in problems in the body. (Also see other lists that precede and follow *Atmospheric Causes*.)

Earth-related Atmospheric Influences

1	Barometric change, weather change, force because of change in altitude
2	Earth gases: ocean, continents (geological decay), radiation
3	Humidity, aridity
4	Hurricane, tornado
5	Lightening storm, rainstorm
6	Sandstorm, ice storm, windstorm, snowstorm
7	Thermal (temperature—cold, hot, warm, cool)
8	Volcanic eruption, earthquake, tidal wave

Cosmic-related Atmospheric Influences

1	Asteroids, meteors, comets
2	Cosmic electrical power
3	Earth changes, planetary/solar system/galaxy/ alignments
4	Gas belts
5	Gravitational pulls
6	Planetary, Big Bang (universe origin)
7	Sunspots

Man-made/Factory-related Atmospheric Influences

1	Chemicals
2	Government release of substances (intentional or unintentional)
3	Manufacturing—industrial, paper, auto
4	Nuclear radiation

People-related Atmospheric Influences

1	Friction (personality, energy fields, polarities)

UFO—Extraterrestrial Influence on the Atmosphere

Continental sources of Atmospheric Influences

1	Africa, Asia, Europe, North America, Australia, South America, Antarctica

Remedies for Atmospheric Influences

- Are there remedies among the following items?
  time, herbs, baths, supplements, physical therapies, other
- There are no remedies.

To Our Health: Using the Inner Art of Dowsing in the Search for Health-Happiness-Harmony in Body-Mind-Spirit

Chemical Causes of Body Issues

Chemicals in the environment can cause body issues. See also *Foods that Can Cause Allergies* p. 43.

Location of Chemical Toxins or Problem Areas

1	Air: factory, utility, natural, man-made
2	Building: home, workplace, school, buildings, church, office
3	Food: farm, factory, home, restaurant
4	Ground: radon gas, minerals, metallic ores, noxious fumes, sand, soil, dirt, clay, land fill
5	Medication: herbal, prescription, over the counter
6	Outdoors site: lake, land, stream, dam, reservoir, construction site
7	Water: ground, well, public water system

Chemicals and Emissions Found Indoors and Outdoors

1	Acids: hydrochloric, sulfuric, ascorbic acid, acetic acid, etc.
2	Clothing/household material: nylon, orlon, polyester, dacron, rayon, polyurethane, acrylic, synthetic, silk, cotton, rami, leather, wool, plastic, rugs, carpets, pads, upholstery, seat cushions, sponge, rubber, pillows, mattress, polyvinyl chloride, sleeping bags
3	Filters: humidifier/dehumidifiers, air conditioner, air purifier, air filters, furnace filters
4	Gaseous emissions: cigarette smoke (from others or self), smokeless tobacco (snuff, chewing), LP gas, butane, lighter fluid (butane), propane, oil furnace, hydrogen fuel, coal tar, machine lubricants
5	Glass: fiberglass insulation and other products
6	Graphics: word processor, printer, computer fumes, fax machines, laminating machines, other office machines
7	Heavy metals: mercury fillings in the mouth; metals in jewelry; mercury, lead, nickel, silver, gold, aluminum, copper, cadmium, tin, plutonium, radium, arsenic, asbestos, strontium 90+; other
8	Paints and stains: varnishes, latex, acrylic, oil, turpentine, paint removers, linseed oil, furniture strippers, wood preservatives, wood stains, etc.
9	Pesticides (insecticides, herbicides, fumigants) or Defoliants: arsenic, DDT, Agent Orange, fungicide
10	Soaps and cleaners: liquid or powder detergents, fabric softener, spot remover, dry cleaning fluid, bleach (chlorine and all fabric), ammonia, mothballs, iron remover, dish washer detergent, water softener
11	Wood: cedar, pine, oak, birch, aspen, beech, poplar, juniper, tamarack, etc.
12	Other: industry-created chemicals, nerve gas, formaldehyde, food irradiation, regular radiation, flame retardant in clothes, carbon monoxide, carbon dioxide

(continued)

Chemical Causes of Body Issues, continued

Personal Care Products

1	Body cleansers and cosmetics: body hair remover, deodorant, antiperspirant, nail polish and remover, creams, conditioners, bubble bath, mouthwash, toothpaste, suppositories, make up, powder, perfume
2	Hair products: permanent wave, shampoo, hair dye, hair spray, hair lightener/darkener
3	Women's sanitary products: tampons, sanitary pads, douche, feminine deodorant spray

Foods and Chemical Additives

1	Caffeine: naturally occurring or added
2	Food additives: BHA, BHT, glycerides, nitrites and nitrates, sulfur dioxide, MSG (monosodium glutamate), benzoyl, peroxide, brominated vegetable oil, EDTA, hydrogenated oils, modified food starch, saccharin, disodium phosphate, sorbitol, dextrin, disodium gecanylate, DES (stilbestrol), potassium sorbate, artificial flavors, colorings, and other additives to food and beverages
3	Food colors: blue dye #1; red dye #2, yellow dye #5, gold, green, purple, orange, brown, or other colors
4	Food kinds: dairy, meat, vegetables, fruit, grain (additives in/or drugs injected into), coffee, chocolate
5	Sodas and alcoholic beverages
6	Sugar: sugar substitutes ("NutraSweet," aspartame, saccharin, sorbitol)
7	Teas
8	Vitamins (see p. 53) and minerals (see p. 53)
9	Other clues: See p. 13 of <u>Additive Book</u> and Hanna Kroeger's <u>God Helps Those That Help Themselves</u>. Please note that additives are being created and added daily to our food.

Drugs and Treatments

1	Drugs - Illegal use, possibly abused or misused: opium, heroin, speed (amphetamines), downers (barbiturates), marijuana (cannabis), cocaine, crack, angel dust, PCP, steroids, inhalants (glues, sprays, other)
2	Medicinal drugs –Over the counter legal drugs: antacid, inhalant, sprays, cold and cough remedies, aspirin, pain killers, laxatives, boric acid, peroxide, alcohol, tobacco
3	Medicinal drugs – Prescription legal drugs: steroids, sleeping pills, hormones, estrogen, tranquilizers, amphetamines, barbiturates, morphine, heart pills, diuretic, blood pressure pills, antibiotics, sprays, inhalants
4	Treatments: dialysis, chemotherapy, radiation, cobalt treatment, chemical therapy
5	Other clues: see prescription and nonprescription drug manuals

Living Things

1	Animals: cats, dogs, birds, deer, rodents, fish, insects, dandruff, feathers, fur, saliva, etc.
2	Chemical sensitivity to people's odor, aura, energy field; to colors; to the sun
3	Microbes: bacteria, viruses, mites, molds, fungi (Candida Albicans, thrush, etc.)
4	Plants
5	Senses: *creation of chemicals because of* sound, taste, fear, touch, sight
6	Sensitivity to people's energies and/or to other's thought pollution; psychic sensitivity

‖ Check other books and references about cause/effects of chemically-induced body issues. ‖

To Our Health: Using the Inner Art of Dowsing in the Search for Health-Happiness-Harmony in Body-Mind-Spirit

Chemical Causes of Body Issues, continued

Ways to Avoid Exposure to Indoor Chemicals

	Indoor Chemical	Ways to Avoid Exposure
1	Alcohols: Rubbing (isopropyl), wood alcohol, ethyl, methyl, spray propellants from astringents, deodorants, depilatories, etc. Paraffins for canning, box coatings.	Avoid fresh paint, varnish and stains. Paint must be non-odorous. No rubber-based paints; casein paints are best. Avoid flavoring extracts.
2	Fuels: Natural gas, coal, heating oil, stove oil, kerosene, wood.	For fuels and cooking use electric heat. Avoid hydrocarbons; gas appliances should be removed from the house, not just disconnected. Remove paints and plastic from heating units.
3	Gasoline and solvents: Lighter fluids, propane, butane, cleaning fluids, ink, ink solvents, marking-pen inks. Adhesives, i.e., glue, tape, bandages. Naphtha, benzene, solvents in detergents and bleaches.	Newspapers and magazines should be aerated before reading. Avoid use of detergents and bleaches; use non-scented soaps. Avoid or replace adhesive in flooring.
4	Pesticides: All insecticides in solid, crystal, or spray form; mothballs; mothproofed clothing; dry cleaning; fumigating agents; fungicides in rubber products.	Avoid rug shampoos that contain DDT. Avoid blankets that are often mothproofed. Aerate clothing after dry-cleaning.
5	Plastics: Toys, plastic bags, vinyl storage containers. Electric-insulating material (heating pads, electric blankets), other insulation, telephones, televisions. Teflon or Silverstone coatings, shower curtains, eye wear. Shoes, insoles.	The more odorous and flexible the plastic, the more likely it will cause symptoms. Allow aeration of plastic products if use cannot be avoided. Have good ventilation when television is in use. Use glass or enamel and cooking containers.
6	Sponge rubber: Pillows, mattresses, rug pads, upholstery, seat cushions.	Use feather pillows or cotton bundles
7	Synthetic fibers: Nylon, acrylic, dacron, polyester, rayon, darnel. Polyurethane (draperies, upholsteries, carpets, bedding).	Wear little synthetic clothing; non-treated cotton is best, undyed wool is good. Do not wear synthetics next to the body.
8	Turpentine and derivatives from pine resins: Paints, paint solvents, cedar chests, odor from Christmas trees, pine-scented household cleaners and fresheners.	(Same as ways to avoid Alcohols, above.)
9	Miscellaneous: Chlorine, ammonia, phenyls, creosol, camphor, methyl. Smoke from natural compounds (tobacco, marijuana, burnt food), perfumes, colognes, scented soaps, cosmetics, sprays. Contraceptives (gels, creams, foams), shaving lotion. Starch, sizing, fabric-treating agents (water repellent, coatings and sprays on outdoor tents or camping equipment).	Avoid tobacco products. Avoid phenyls and other chemicals that are in wallpaper paste; purchase natural-based paste. Silver and brass polishing compounds contain toxic fumes; use baking soda instead.

Cosmic, Celestial, Planet Earth Influences and Their Resolutions

Cosmic phenomena, influences from celestial bodies, earth seasons and weather phenomena can cause body issues.

Cosmic and Celestial Influences

Column 1	Column 2	Column 3	Column 4	Column 5
• Astrology	• Astronomy	• Black hole	• Comets	• Constellations
• Cosmic rays	• Galaxies	• Gravity	• Heaven	• Meteors
• Nebula	• Planets	• Star brightness	• Star clusters	• Star distance
• Star light	• Stars	• Universal energies		
• Moon	• Lunar calendar	• Lunar halo	• Lunar eclipse	
• Solar system	• Solar eclipse	• Van Allen belt	• Solar wind—faster near the sun's pole	
• Sun	• Solar flares	• Sunlight	• Sunspots	

Planet Earth Influences

Column 1	Column 2	Column 3
• Rainbows	• Magnetic field reflects the northern/southern lights	• Tidal influences
• Earth motion		• Tides
• Equinox—spring or fall	• Auroras (northern/southern lights)	• Sunrise
• Solstice—summer or winter	• Day/night	• Sunset
• Altitude—high or low	• Earth circulation	• Season
• El Nino effect	• El Nina effect	• Climate
• Atmosphere	• Dampness/humidity	• Temperature
• Hurricanes	• Tornadoes	• Rainfall
• Frost	• Snow	• Squall lines
• Winds	• Clouds: nimbus, cumulus, stratus, etc.	• Hail
• Air masses: polar, tropical, warm, cold, high pressure, low pressure	• Blotchball effect—atmospheric force	• Storms: lightening, ice storms, thunderstorms

Resolutions for Cosmic, Celestial, and Planet Earth Influences

- One needs to find one's place or purpose in the universe.
- Practice conscious control or effect on weather (e.g.-cloud busting).
- Be aware of weather patterns and weather changes.
- Pay close attention to planetary and cosmic motions.
- Notice that one is strongly influenced by celestial or planetary motions and occurrences.
- Do/do not focus on planetary/cosmic influences.

Electrical, Polar, Gravitational Influences and Their Resolutions

(Also Electromagnetic Influences)

Electrical, Polar, Gravitational, and Electromagnetic Influences

1	Wiring Car vehicle Car batteries Submarine Train Airplane Transmitters Receivers
2	Electrical power plant Substations High-power lines Gridding Grid lines
3	Computer lines Computer terminal Communication, government
4	Corporate satellites–surveillance, weather Microwave transmitters
5	CB Radio waves Radar—high frequency Radio broadcast
6	Laser Ultraviolet rays Ultraviolet light Cosmic rays Infrared light Infrared camera
7	Sunspot season—will affect radio, TV, people, etc. Static Lightening
8	Energy vortex—noxious, positive
9	Electromagnetic null zone—energy vacuum where there is an absence of electromagnetic fields
10	Van Allen belt (energy pattern that flows around the earth)
11	Copier Photocopier FAX machine Labeler Power tools
12	Newspaper bundler Electric wiring in the home Alarm clock Coffee pot
13	Electric blanket Heating pad Water bed heater
14	Electric stove Dryers Washers VCR Television Microwave
15	Hot water heater Garage door opener Remote controls Watch/ batteries
16	Vibration of any kind of toothbrush, shaver, water pick
17	Light bulbs: neon, tanning lights, incandescent, growing/growlight bulbs, florescent lighting, dimmer, 3-way bulbs, night light, other lights
18	Light emitting diodes (LED)
19	Phone company Phones: mobile, cellular, digital, rotary, push button, touch tone, pulse tone
20	Video games: home, arcade, hand-held Low/high frequency electrical vibrations
21	Ley lines on the earth: noxious, positive Earth's polarity Gravitational influences
22	UFO/extraterrestrial influence Aura Chakras
23	Body energy Axiational energy lines Electrical friction between people
24	Electromagnetic wave (telepathy/psychic energy) Electrical short circuit in the body or auric field
25	Magnetic or electric interference with the body, mind, spirit functions

Resolutions to Balance Electrical and Related Influences

- Walk barefoot on wet grass.
- Remove/avoid/use formulas, tinctures, teas (rosemary), etc.
- Wear wool.
- Wear silk.
- Wear or touch a multipole magnet to stimulate the body and help control electricity in your body.
- Hug a tree to balance electromagnetic field in oneself. Cherry and poplar are most beneficial.
- Use both hands to grasp a metal post or kitchen faucet.

Environmental Influences and Their Resolutions

These may be cross-referenced with the following influences: *Atmospheric* p. 44; *Chemical* p. 45; *Cosmic, Celestial, Planet Earth* p. 48; *Physical* p. 54; *Emotional* pp. 56 and 57; *Spiritual* p. 68; and *Social* p. 95.

Environmental Influences

1	Air Water Ground Ozone Dust Radon Alpha waves Radiation Metallic poisons
2	Foods Moon Tide Wind Ley lines Nuclear fallout Radioactive decay
3	Medication Minerals (see *Minerals* p. 53) Elements (check *Elements from Periodic Table*, below)
4	Influence from others Thought pollution Neglect
5	Animals: domesticated pets, wildlife, birds Animal-borne diseases
6	Insects: roaches, fleas, mites (indoor/outdoor), ticks Pests and parasites
7	Plants: molds, fungus, house plants, pollen
8	Microbes: bacteria, virus, viroid, worms, parasites, amoebas

Elements, from Periodic Table, That Can Influence Body Issues

The following elements are found in various forms—gases or solids or liquids.

1	Hydrogen Helium Lithium Beryllium Boron Carbon Nitrogen Oxygen Fluorine Neon Sodium
2	Magnesium Aluminum Silicon Phosphorus Sulfur Chlorine Argon Potassium Calcium Scandium
3	Titanium Vanadium Chromium Manganese Iron Cobalt Nickel Copper Zinc Gallium Germanium
4	Arsenic Selenium Bromine Krypton Rubidium Strontium Yttrium Zirconium Niobium
5	Molybdenum *Technetium Ruthenium Rhodium Palladium Silver Cadmium Indium Tin
6	Antimony Tellurium Iodine Xenon Cesium Barium Lanthanum Hafnium Tantalum Tungsten
7	Rhenium Osmium Iridium Platinum Gold Mercury Thallium Lead Bismuth Polonium
8	Astatine Radon Francium Radium Actinium Cerium Praseodymium Neodymium
9	*Promethium Samarium Europium Gadolinium Terbium Dysprosium Holmium
10	Erbium Thulium Ytterbium Lutetium Thorium Protactinium Uranium *Neptunium
11	*Plutonium *Americium *Curium *Berkelium *Californium *Einsteinium *Fermium
12	*Mendelevium *Nobelium *Lawrencium *Unnilquadium *Unnilpentium *Unnilhexium

(*** = man-made elements**)

Possible Resolutions of Environmental Influences

- Clean the home/space.
- One needs to leave the environment.
- Restructure the environment.
- Clean up the environment.
- One's environmental interaction with others needs modification.
- Use tinctures, formulas, supplements, etc. to counteract environmental influences.
- One needs to resolve being bothered by living in the environment, for example:
  - One is bothered by the way the environment looks, smells, or feels.
  - Memories or patterns were left behind by former occupants.
  - Environment is not suitable for health/well-being.

Nutritional Influences and Their Resolutions

Nutritional deficiencies, excesses, contamination, and imbalances can cause body issues.

Deficiencies or Excesses in Nutrition

Column 1	Column 2	Column 3	Column 4
• Acid-alkaline balance	• Amino acids	• Aroma	• Carbohydrates
• Dairy products	• Enzymes	• Fats	• Food supplements
• Fruits	• Grain	• Herbs	• Minerals
• Proteins: meats, nuts, seeds	• Sodium/potassium balance	• Spices	• Taste
• Teas	• Tinctures	• Vegetables	• Vitamins
• Water			

Resolutions for Deficiencies or Excess

- Check the following lists: *Foods that Can Cause Allergies* p. 43; *Vitamins* p. 53, and *Minerals* p. 53.
- Check for allergies, physical disorder, chemical disorder, anorexia, and bulimia.
- Check for proper ingestion/absorption, digestion/excretion, muscle/fat ratio, caloric intake, food combination.
- Check time of day for taking food: too early or too late.
- Check for quantity: too much or not enough.
- Check for suitability: should eat a food or should not eat it.
- Check for reactive eating—stress-related eating patterns associated with family, friends, job, etc.
- Check for kind of nutrition needed, for example:
  - Nutrition obtained by being in the company of friends, family or other relatives, teachers
  - Need food that's freshly prepared and cooked
- Is the environment, in which one takes in nutrition, healthy?
  - Physical environment: clubs, workplace, restaurant, home, school
  - How and when one eats
  - Mental and spiritual environment
- One needs to: relax   hurry   eat together   eat apart.
- Some nutrients are contaminated with   bacteria   chemicals   radiation
- Consider fasting (juice, water, etc.).
- Change one's diet.

Nutritional Influences and Resolutions, continued

Acid-Alkaline Balance

A proper acid-alkaline balance in our body is important to maintenance of health. Our bodies try to maintain a slightly alkaline pH of 7.4. (The pH scale ranges from 1 to 14, 7.0 being neutral. Anything below 7.0 is acidic, while anything above 7.0 is alkaline.) With proper acid-alkaline balance, there is an electronic balance of ions or charged particles in the bloodstream. According to Edgar Cayce, the body will stay balanced when one consumes 80 percent alkaline-producing food and 20 percent acid-producing food.

Examples of Acid-Producing Foods

1	bacon barley beef: corned, dried, liver, porterhouse, round, sirloin	bread, white
2	buckwheat cheddar cheese chicken, broilers codfish, salt corn, canned cornmeal	
3	crackers, soda eggs, whole frog's legs haddock halibut ham, smoked	
4	lamb, leg lentils mackerel, fresh and salt mutton, leg oatmeal, rolled	
5	oysters pork chops rice salmon sardines sausage shredded wheat	
6	turkey veal, leg walnuts wheat, cracked whitefish	

Examples of Alkaline-Producing Foods

Note: this is not a complete list

1	almonds apples apricots asparagus bananas			
2	beans: baked, dried kidney, dried, lima, canned, string	beets, fresh	buttermilk	cabbage
3	carrots cauliflower celery chard	cherries	chestnuts	cream
4	cucumbers dates figs, dried grapes	grape juice	lemons	lettuce
5	milk: whole and skim molasses olives	onions	oranges	
6	orange juice parsnips peaches, fresh/canned	pears, canned	pineapple	
7	potatoes pumpkins radishes raisins	rhubarb	spinach	
8	squash tomatoes turnips watermelons			

Resolution: Eat Foods to Restore Acid-Alkaline Balance

- Charcoal—eat a burnt piece of toast to counteract food poisoning or diarrhea or to balance stomach acid.
- Eat Alka-thyme product to balance acid-alkaline levels in the body.

Resolution: Avoid Eating Certain Foods Together

- Two or more starchy foods at the same meal
- Sugary foods and starchy
- Milk and citrus fruit or juice
- Citrus fruit or juice and cereals
- Starchy foods with meat or cheese
- Coffee with milk or cream
- Raw apples with other food

Nutritional Influences and Resolutions, continued

Vitamins

- A (retinol, beta carotene)
- B-1 (thiamine)
- B-3 (niacin)
- B-6 (pyridoxine)
- B-17 (laetrile)
- D (D-2 or calciferol, D-3 in fish liver oils)
- F (unsaturated fatty acids, linoleic, linolenic, oleic)
- P (bioflavonoids, vitamin P citrin, flavonals, flavones, hesperidin, rutin)

- B complex: biotin, choline, folic acid-folacin, inositol, pantothenic acid
- B-2 (riboflavin)
- B-5 (pantothenic Acid)
- B-12 (cobalamin)
- C (ascorbic acid)
- E (tocopherol, d'alpha, dl'alpha, tocopheryl)
- K (menadione)
- PABA (para-aminobenzoic acid)

Minerals

- Boron
- Cobalt
- Chlorine
- Fluorine
- Iodine
- Magnesium
- Molybdenum
- Potassium
- Silicon (Silica)
- Sulfur
- Zinc

- Calcium
- Chromium
- Copper
- Germanium
- Iron
- Manganese
- Phosphorus
- Selenium
- Sodium
- Vanadium

Amino Acids

- L-Alanine
- L-Asparagine
- L-Carnitine
- L-Cysteine
- Gamma-aminobutyric acid
- L-Glutamine
- L-Glycine
- L-Isoleucine
- L-Lysine
- L-Ornithine
- DL-Phenylalanine
- L-Serine
- L-Tryptophan
- L-Tyrosine

- L-Arginine
- L-Aspartic acid
- L-Citrulline
- L-Cystine
- L-Glutamic acid
- L-Glutathione
- L-Histidine
- L-Leucine
- L-Methionine
- L-Phenylalanine
- L-Proline
- L-Taurine
- L-Threonine
- L-Valine

Enzymes

Enzymes are formed from proteins. There are millions of enzymes. Many are produced by the body, and others are available from raw (uncooked) foods. See examples below.

1	Amylase	Bromelain	Catalase	Chymotrypsin	Lipase
2	Pancreatin	Papain	Superoxide dismutase	Trypsin	

Proteins, Carbohydrates, and Fats

See books about nutrition for more about effect of dietary proteins, carbohydrates, and fats on the body.

Physical Influences

Influences listed here may come up when working on the *Body Chart* p. 17 or on step 6 *How is issue manifested on/in/around the body?* for the *Out of Balance Checklist.*

Also see the following influences, which may be related to Physical influences: *Symptoms of Food Allergies and Other Allergies* p. 42, *Chemical Causes of Body Issues* p. 45, *Nutritional Issues and Resolutions* p. 51, and lists that follow *Physical Issues.*

> There are many corresponding factors that might be manifested physically. Check medical, spiritual, emotional, holistic, and other reference materials.

Physical Events that Might Cause the Issue

Abuse	Accident	Dis-ease	Misuse	Neglect	Operation	Shock	Trauma

How or Where Is the Issue Manifested in the Body?

1	See Hanna Kroeger's book <u>Seven Spiritual Causes of Ill Health</u>
2	Blood disturbance
3	Genetic: RNA or DNA disturbance
4	Immune system imbalance
5	Inherited disease
6	Nutrition: over eating, undereating, imbalanced diet, improper food combination, lacking vitamins, lacking minerals, insufficient water (dehydration), excesses (vitamins, minerals, coffee, etc.), acid-alkaline imbalance
7	Nervous system: autonomic, sympathetic, parasympathetic
8	Skin: the body's envelope is being affected
9	Cellular disorder: cancer or pre-cancer condition
10	Miasma: carried-over disease, genetic—origin is long ago, for example four or five generations ago
11	Inoculations: left undesirable residue (tetanus, NIRI, diphtheria, rubella, mumps, measles, undisclosed, etc.)
12	Tuberculosis: scoliosis, hammertoe, bunions, enlarged painful finger joints, arthritis. (Generally, Miasma come in with weak lungs but hardly ever manifest in the body as tuberculosis.)
13	Sexually transmitted diseases: syphilis, gonorrhea, chlamydia, AIDS or HIV, etc.
14	Headaches: muscle spasm brings on tension headaches; vascular changes can cause a headache when blood vessels dilate in the brain; migraine and cluster (vascular); organic causes (tumors or infection) of headaches are rare
15	Infections or congestion: staphylococcus, streptococcus, other bacterial infections, thrush or other Candida Albicans infection, virus, viroid, ebola, Epstein-Barr, etc.
16	Parasites: parasitic worms, parasites carried by ticks (Rocky Mt. Fever, Lyme disease). (Note: Baylisascaris procyonis is carried by raccoons and is highly dangerous.) (See Hanna Kroeger book in *References.*)
17	Animal or insect sources: bites, feces, urine, fur, eggs, skin, blood, meats, sperm, saliva
18	Biorhythm disturbances: physical, mental, emotional cycles
19	Body cycles: male cycles, female cycles (menstruation, menopause)

(continued)

Physical Issues, continued

Brain's Four Layers
- The first layer, the ancient layer, gives territorialism and survival mechanisms.
- The second layer, the early human brain, is the home of our emotions, motivation, feelings, limbic system.
- The third layer, the modern brain, consists of right and left lobes (hemispheres) that provide thinking, creativity, memorization, inventiveness, realization, and judging.
- The fourth layer, the developing brain (a new layer that is at present in the process of developing), is the source of intelligence, intuition, compassion, consciousness, and has unlimited potential for receiving information.

Childhood Diseases, Resolutions and Preventive Measures

Listed below are diseases occurring in childhood that can cause body issues.

Column 1	Column 2
• Accidents and poisoning	• Allergy
• Contagious diseases	• Disease of the blood
• Gastrointestinal disease	• Genito-urinary disease
• Heart disease	• Infectious diseases
• Muscle disease	• Neurologic conditions of childhood
• Orthopedic conditions	• Skeletal disease
• Surgical condition of the abdomen	• Uncommon disease in newborn

Listed below are common resolutions and preventive measures for childhood diseases.

• Antibiotics	• Pain medication, cold and cough medication
• Fluoride treatment, toothpastes	• Vitamins and minerals

Imprinting during Conception, while a Person Was in the Womb, or at Birth

Column 1	Column 2
• Emotional imprint	• Mental/intellectual imprint
• Physical imprint	• Spiritual imprint
• Genetic family imprint (past experience in family tree hangs over as a *Dark Cloud*)	

Other Manifestations in This Organ or Body Part

Column 1	Column 2
• Exhausted	• Got a foreign object
• Hyperactive	• Hypoactive
• Inflamed	• Malfunctioning
• Overexerted	• Overextended
• Overworked	• Stagnant
• Underworked	

INFLUENCES ON MIND ISSUES

Table of Contents

Emotional Gauge for HHH Dowsing

These energies or emotions can be created by yourself or by others. Find the most important positive energy and negative energy on this page for an issue. Also see additional *Negative Words* p. 58, additional *Positive Words* p. 63, and *Chakras* p. 73.

Positive Energy	Chakra Relates to Color and Attitude	Negative Energy
Determination Expect Hugging Onward Provide Seeking Truth and wholeness Wish	**Neo Brain** (above the Crown chakra) Transparent Clearing 8	Cast out Framed Inferior Irritated Lazy (Too) outspoken Speak out/up
Absolute Assurance At-one-ment Bliss Brand new Correct Encouraged Erect Expecting Involved Perfect	**Crown** White Appreciation 7	Behind Confused Encircled Fuming Loses Not listened to Pointed Pride Ruined Surprised Tight Youngster (immaturity)
Aware Buoyancy Comparable Determination Erect In tune Pride Relief	**Brow** Indigo Admiration 6	Encumbered Faded Left out Mean Resolved Tight Troubled Unselfish Vulgar Youngster (immaturity)
Abstain Assurance Beautiful Best Change Enjoy Fulfilled Involved Moving Precious Sign Simple Speak out/up (Too) outspoken Turn	**Throat** Blue Willing 5	Bold Challenged Directed Evoked Forgetting Hustled Intrenched Loveless Morbid Not generous Oppressed Outspoken Tempted Transgressed
Abstain Accommodate Attainment Buoyancy Clearing Compassion Compassionate Determination Divine Expect Loving Moving Perfect Precise Support Writing Youngster (immaturity)	**Heart** Green Attunement 4	Abject Embarrassed Emptiness Grumbling Hitched Introverted Morbid Persecuted Possessed Queer Rigid Rotted Stinky Yanking Youngster (immaturity)
Accomplish Adjusted Attuned Changeable Channel Coexist Decision Employ Enchantment Engaging Erect In tune Loving place Slender Turn	**Solar Plexus** Yellow Assurance 3	Antagonism Bribed Confused Defeated Depressed Evoked Frightened Frustrated Paralyzed
Acceptance Acquit Attuned Clearing Climbing Collected Delightful Elated Enfold Frugal Godly Knowing myself In time Precious Surprise Transition Wonder	**Sex** Orange Interest 2	Conquered Depressed Entangled Frightened Fuming Indifferent Loaded down Overreact Reform Seeking Void Zoned
Changeable Choosing Dynamic Employ Encouragement Enfold Godly Knowing Lord Peace Place Stability Trust	**Root** Red Oneness 1	Bereaved Conceited Humiliated Lied about or lied to Overcharged Oversensitive Rejected Sorry for self Trapped Troubled

Negative Emotional Influences and Resolutions

‖ Fear in your mind produces fear in your life in Body-Mind-Spirit. This is the meaning of hell! ‖

‖ You live on borrowed or chosen emotions at times. ‖

For additional clues, see *Physical Influences* p. 54; *Chemical Causes* p. 45; *Mental or Intellectual Influences* p. 66; and various influences listed in the *Table of Contents* p. 86 for *Body-Mind-Spirit Issues.*

Possible Negative Events

Did one of the following events influence the issue?

Abuse	Accident	Dis-ease	Misuse	Neglect	Operation	Shock	Trauma

What Is the Source of the Negative Emotional Influence?

Self   Other(s)   Situation

Negative Words that May Represent How the Body-Mind-Spirit Feels

Column 1	Column 2	Column 3	Column 4	Column 5
• Aback	• Abatement	• Abandoned	• Abasement	• Abashment
• Abdication	• Abduction	• Abet	• Abeyance	• Abhorrent
• Abiding	• Abject	• Able	• Abnormal	• Abolished
• Abomination	• Aboriginal	• Abortive	• Abrupt	
• Abuse: emotional, physical, mental, sexual, spiritual, financial				
• Accountable	• Accursed	• Accusing	• Acrid	• Adventurous
• Affectionate	• Agitated	• Anger	• Annoyed	• Antagonism
• Anxiety	• Anxious	• Assured	• At fault	• Attacked
• Backstabb(ing, ed)	• Bad	• Bad loser	• Balking	• Batter(ed, -ing)
• Bearing	• Beaten	• Belligerent	• Begrudge	• Beguiled
• Behind	• Bereaved	• Beseeched	• Betrayed	• Bewildered
• Beyond	• Bitter	• Boredom	• Bold	• Bothered
• Bypasses				
• Calm	• Capricious	• Captured	• Cast out	• Castaway
• Caught	• Cautious	• Challenged	• Cheap	• Cheated
• Choked	• Clinging	• Cluttered	• Compulsive	• Conceited
• Concerned	• Conflict	• Confused	• Conquered	• Conspiring
• Contemptible	• Costly	• Countless	• Crazed or crazy	• Creative
• Critical	• Cross	• Crouching	• Cynicism	

(continued)

Negative Emotional Influences, continued

Column 1	Column 2	Column 3	Column 4	Column 5
• Dead end	• Decrepit	• Defeated	• Depressed	• Deprived
• Deserted	• Destructive	• Detailed	• Diligent	• Directed
• Disappointed	• Disciplined	• Disconnected	• Discontent	• Discontented
• Discouraged	• Disguised	• Disharmony	• Dishonest	• Dislike(d)
• Disloyal	• Distracted	• Distressed	• Disunited	• Dominant
• Dominated	• Doubt	• Dread	• Dumb (mute or unintelligent)	
• Egocentric	• Egoless	• Egotistical	• Eliminated	• Eluding
• Embarrassed	• Embittered	• Empathy	• Emptiness	• Encircled
• Encountered	• Encumbered	• Endangered	• Endowed	• Enslaved
• Entangled	• Enticed	• Envy	• Erased	• Erratic
• Esoteric	• Evocative	• Evoked	• Exasperated	• Exhausted
• Eye for detail	• Eye for an eye			
• Facetious	• Faded	• Failure	• Fair	• Fear
• Feeble	• Festering	• Fickle	• Fiery	• Filthy
• Fixed	• Forceful	• Forcible	• Forgetting	• Forgiven
• Forgiving	• Forlorn	• Formidable	• Foul	• Framed
• Free(ing)	• Friction	• Frightened	• Frigid	• Frustrated
• Fuming	• Fundamentalist	• Furious	• Fused	• Fussy
• Futile				
• Gaudy	• Gawking	• Ghastly	• Giddy	• Gimmicky
• Gossipy	• Greedy	• Grief for others or for self	• Grievance	• Griping
• Gripping	• Grouchy	• Goaded	• Grudge	• Grumbling
• Guilt	• Gut feeling			
• Hard	• Harmful	• Hate	• Haughty	• Haunted
• Heaviness	• Heckled	• Helpless	• Hesitant	• Hindered
• Hitched	• Hoax	• Holding on	• Hopeless	• Horrible
• Hostile	• Humiliation	• Humorless	• Humorous	• Hurried
• Hurt	• Hustled	• Hysterical		
• Ignored	• Imaginative	• Immaterial	• Immobilized	• Impatient
• Impulsive	• Inadequate	• Incensed	• Inconvenienced	• Indifferent
• Indignant	• Individualistic	• Indomitable	• Indulged	• Inebriated
• Ineffective	• Ineligible	• Inert	• Inexpressible	• Inferior
• Inflated ego	• Injustice	• Inner-direction	• Insecure	• Insensitive
• Intelligent	• Intercepted	• Intolerant	• Introverted	• Intruded upon
• Irresistible	• Irritant	• Irritated		

(continued)

Negative Emotional Influences, continued

Column 1	Column 2	Column 3	Column 4	Column 5
• Jammed	• Jealous	• Jeopardized	• Joking	• Jumpy
• Justice	• Justified			
• Kind	• Kinship	• Knifed	• Knocked down	• Knotted
• Know-it-all	• Knowledgeable			
• Lack of	• Lassitude	• Lazy	• Least	• Leaving
• Left out	• Less	• Let down	• Liable	• Lied about
• Lied for	• Lied to	• Lifeless	• Limited	• Listless
• Live in fantasy	• Living in past	• Load is too heavy or big or small	• Loaded down	• Lonely
• Loser	• Loss	• Lost	• Loveless	• Lower
• Mad (angry, crazy)	• Mangled	• Marked	• Martyr	• Masked
• Materialistic	• Mean	• Melancholy	• Merciless	• Meticulous
• Minced	• Mindless	• Misappreciated	• Misappropriated	• Misbelief
• Misconduct	• Miser	• Miserable	• Miserly	• Misfit
• Misjudged	• Mistrust	• Misunderstood or misunderstanding	• Moody	• Morbid
• Neglected	• Nervous	• No end	• No faith in future	• No love for/ from self or others
• Noisy	• Nonexistence	• Nonmaterialistic	• Not functioning	• Not generous
• Not happy	• Not heard	• Not liked	• Not liking self	• Not listened to
• Not listening	• Not taken (taking) care of	• Not understood	• Not liking others	• Numb
			• Noxious	
• Obnoxious	• Obsession	• Obstruct(ed)	• Odd	• Off
• Offended	• Opposing	• Oppressed	• Orgasmic	• Out of balance
• Out of tune	• Outraged	• Outspoken	• Overact	• Overburdened
• Overcharge(d)	• Overloaded	• Overlooked	• Overreact	• Oversensitive
• Overtake(n)	• Overtired	• Overweight	• Overwhelmed	• Overworked
• Overwrought				
• Pain	• Panic	• Paralyzed	• Parting	• Passed
• Pathetic	• Patrol(ed/ing)	• Patroniz(ing/ed)	• Peculiar	• Permissive
• Persecuted	• Perturbed	• Perverted	• Pessimistic	• Petrified
• Picked on	• Picky	• Pitied	• Pitiful	• Pity
• Plagued	• Plain	• Playful	• Pointed	• Poised
• Poisoned	• Political	• Pollut(ed/er)	• Positive	• Possessed

(continued)

Negative Emotional Influences, continued

Column 1	Column 2	Column 3	Column 4	Column 5
Possessive	Power(ful/less)	Present	Preserv(ed/ing)	Pressed upon
Pressing	Pretending	Prevailed upon	Prevailing	Prevent(ed/ive)
Progressive	Prohibited	Promised	Prosecuted	Proud
Provincial	Provocative	Psychic	Pugnacious	Punished
Pursued	Put down	Put off/put on	Put upon	Putrid
Quaking	Quandary (in a)	Quarrelsome	Queasy	Queer
Quenched	Querying	Questioned	Questioning	Quiet
Quip	Quitter	Quitting		
Racial	Rage	Rationalist	Realistic	Reaping
Rebuffed	Reckless	Reclining	Reclusive	Restrained
Reconverted	Recurring	Reflecting	Reflecting	Reflective
Rejected	Released	Releasing	Religious	Repentant
Repetitious	Reposed	Reproached	Reproachment	Resented
Resentful	Resentful	Resentment	Resigned	Resolved
Restless	Retribution	Revenge	Rigid	Rotted
Rough	Rude	Rudimentary	Ruined	Rut
Sacrificing	Sad	Sarcastic	Sassy	Satisfied
Saturated	Screaming	Searching	See no end	See not
Seeing	Seeking	Seething	Self esteem	Self-effacing
Self-empowered	Self-love	Self-pity	Self-punishment	Self-worth
Sensitive	Sentimental	Separation	Shy	Silly
Sitter	Sitting out	Situational	Skinny	Smiling
Smothered	Smothering	Soaring	Sober	Soothing
Sordid	Sorrow	Sorry for self or others	Sorting	Speak out
Speechless	Spiteful	Spongy	Spontaneous	Squandering
Squelching	Stagnant	Sticky	Stingy	Stinky
Stirring	Stressed	Strong / strong willed	Struggling	Stubborn
Stuck-up	Stupid	Stuttering	Suffering	Suffragette
Suitable	Sullen	Surfacing	Symbolic	Sympathetic
Taken	Talented	Tantrum	Tattletale	Taught
Teaching	Tempted	Tenacious	Terror	Thin
Thorough	Thoughtful	Thoughtless	Threatened	Thrifty
Thrilled	Through	Thrown away	Tight	Timid
Tortured	Tough	Toxic	Tragic	Transgressed
Transgressor	Trapped	Tribulation	Trick(ed, y)	Troubled
Trusting	Trustworthy	Trusty	Turned in or turn upon	

(continued)

Negative Emotional Influences, continued

Column 1	Column 2	Column 3	Column 4	Column 5
• Unacceptable	• Unaccepted	• Unafraid	• Unappreciated	• Uncaring
• Uncontrollable	• Uncontrollable	• Unconventional	• Uncooperative	• Uncourageous
• Underage	• Underfed	• Underlined	• Undernourished	• Undertaken
• Undeserving	• Undesirable	• Undetermined	• Uneasy	• Uneducated
• Unengaged	• Unfair	• Unfolding	• Unforeseen	• Unforgiven
• Unforgiving	• Unfulfilled	• Unfulfilling	• Ungiving	• Unhappy
• Unheard	• Unimportant	• Unknown	• Unlovable	• Unloved
• Unnoticed	• Unorthodox	• Unreadable	• Unrealistic	• Unreliable
• Unresponsive	• Unseen	• Unsolvable	• Unstable	• Unsubmissive
• Unsupportive	• Unsympathetic	• Untold	• Unusual	• Unwelcome
• Unwilling	• Urged	• Usable	• Used	• Useless
• Using	• Utilizing			
• Vague	• Vain	• Valueless	• Vengeance	• Venture
• Vicious	• Villain	• Vindicated	• Vindicating	• Vindictive
• Violat(ed, ing)	• Violent	• Virulent	• Void	• Voluptuous
• Voracious	• Vulgar			
• X-rated	• Xenobiotic	• Xenogeneic	• Xenophobic	• Xerophilous
• Yabbering	• Yacking	• Yammering	• Yanking	• Yapping
• Yawning	• Yawping	• Yearning	• Yech	• Yelling
• Yelping	• Yen	• Yes-man	• Yielding	• Yodeling
• Yogic	• Yoked	• Yoo-hoo	• Yore	• Young(er, est)
• Youngster (immature)	• Yourself	• Youth	• Yowling	• Yucky
				• Yuppie
• Zany	• Zapped	• Zealot	• Zealous	• Zero
• Zombie	• Zoned	• Zonked		

Resolutions for Mind Issues Caused by Negative Emotional Influences

- See *Emotional Gauge for HHH Dowsing* p. 57.
- See one or more of the following: counselor, psychiatrist, psychologist, 12-step programs.
- Engage in exercise and other physical activities—action—pinching (a pillow), punching (a pillow), running, walking, pillow fighting, running away, or confronting others.
- Voice—crying, screaming, singing, talking, listening.
- Creativity—drawing, painting, writing, reading.
- Check for—lack of sleep, food, nutrition.
- Check *Resolutions* p. 105.
- Also check through appropriate books and literature.

Positive Words, Statements, and Feelings

This is how your Body-Mind-Spirit truly wants to feel.

Column 1	Column 2	Column 3	Column 4	Column 5
• Abide	• Ability	• Able	• Abound	• Above
• Absolute	• Absolve	• Abstain	• Abundance	• Acceptance
• Acclaim	• Accommodate	• Accompaniment	• Accomplish	• Accord
• Accredit	• Accrue	• Accurate	• Achieve	• Acknowledgment
• Acquaint	• Acquire	• Acquit	• Act	• Active
• Actual	• Adaptable	• Add	• Adequate	• Adhere
• Adjust	• Admirable	• Admissible	• Adopt	• Adorable
• Adorn	• Adventurous	• Affair	• Affectionate	• Afloat
• Aggrandize	• Aggrandize	• Alight	• Align	• Alike
• Alive	• Allot	• Ambitious	• Amused	• Amusement
• Angelic	• Appease	• Appreciated	• Approachable	• Artistic
• Assurance	• Assured	• At peace	• Atonement	• Attractive
• Attuned	• Available	• Aware		
• Balance	• Beautiful	• Become	• Best	• Blend
• Bliss	• Bold	• Brand new	• Buoyancy	• Buoyed
• Busy				
• Called on	• Calm	• Caring	• Celebrate	• Certain
• Challenge	• Change(d)	• Changeable	• Channel	• Choosing
• Circulating	• Clearing	• Climbing	• Coexist	• Cognition
• Cognizable	• Collaborate	• Collected	• Comfortable	• Committed
• Communicate	• Comparable	• Compassion	• Compatible	• Compensate
• Complete	• Complete	• Compliment	• Compose	• Comradery
• Conceptualizing	• Concerned	• Connected	• Considered	• Consistent
• Consolidate	• Constancy	• Consultative	• Content	• Contribute
• Convenience	• Conventional	• Conversant	• Cooperative	• Cope
• Correct	• Creative			
• Daring	• Decide	• Decision	• Delightful	• Dependable
• Deserving	• Determination	• Different	• Divine	• Dynamic
• Efficient	• Elated	• Elevated	• Emerging	• Employ
• Empower	• Enchantment	• Encouragement	• Endeavor	• Endurance
• Enfold	• Engaging	• Enhance	• Enjoy	• Enlighten
• Enter	• Enthusiasm	• Equal	• Erect	• Essential
• Esteem	• Eternal	• Ever	• Excel	• Excepting
• Excited	• Expect			

(continued)

Positive Words, Statements, and Feelings, continued

Column 1	Column 2	Column 3	Column 4	Column 5
• Fabulous	• Faith	• Fantastic	• Fidelity	• Flexibility
• Flourish	• Forgo	• Forthcoming	• Fortunate	• Forward
• Frugal	• Fulfilled	• Future		
• Gentle	• Giving	• God Force	• Godly	• Gratuitous
• Guidance	• Guided			
• Handling	• Heal	• Heartfelt	• High	• Honest
• Hugging				
• Illuminated	• Illustrating	• Imperishable	• Improving	• In balance
• Increase	• In tune	• Infinite	• Innermost	• Innocence
• Innovation	• Interested	• Involved	• Irradiant	• Itself
• Jolly	• Joy			
• Kind	• Kindly	• Knowing	• Known	
• Leisure	• Light	• Lightened	• Lord	• Love
• Lovely	• Loving	• Lyrical		
• Manifest	• Mediate	• Meditate	• Mellow	• Mindful
• Motivate	• Moving	• Myself	• Mystic	
• Needed	• Negotiate	• Nominal	• Normal	
• Observable	• Oneness	• Oneself	• Onward	• Open
• Outreach	• Overt			
• Parley	• Passion	• Peace	• Perceptive	• Perfect
• Perseverance	• Place	• Play	• Please	• Pleasure
• Pledge	• Plentiful	• Poise	• Portray	• Positive
• Possibility	• Practicable	• Practice	• Praise	• Prayer
• Precede	• Precious	• Prefer	• Prepare	• Prepossess
• Presence	• Present	• Preserve	• Prestige	• Pride
• Productive	• Prosper	• Protected	• Proud	• Provide
• Purpose	• Put			

(continued)

Positive Words, Statements, and Feelings, continued

Column 1	Column 2	Column 3	Column 4	Column 5
• Quick	• Quiet	• Quoting		
• Radiant	• Radiate	• Rate	• Reach	• Realm
• Reason	• Reassure	• Receivable	• Receptive	• Reeducate
• Reestablish	• Refill	• Refine	• Reflect	• Reform
• Refresh	• Regard	• Rejoice	• Relate	• Relax
• Release	• Relevant	• Relief	• Relieve	• Rely
• Remark	• Remind	• Render	• Replace	• Replenish
• Repose	• Request	• Require	• Research	• Reserve
• Respect	• Reunification	• Review	• Rise	• Romance
• Satisfactory	• Seer	• Select	• Sensibility	• Serve
• Share	• Sign	• Signal	• Simple	• Sincere
• Skillful	• Slender	• Smart	• Sophisticated	• Sound
• Sovereign	• Spontaneous	• Stability	• Stern	• Strength
• Suggest	• Support	• Surprise	• Swept away	• System
• Talent	• Task	• Team	• Tender	• Thanks
• Tidy	• Together	• Total	• Touch	• Transform
• Transition	• Triumph	• True	• Trust	• Truth
• Turn	• Twinkle			
• Unify	• Union	• Unison	• Unit	• Universe
• Unselfish	• Unshaken	• Up	• Urge	• Utter
• Venture	• Virtuous	• Vision	• Visionary	
• Warrior	• Welcome	• Wholeness	• Willing	• Winning
• Wish	• Won	• Wonder	• Writing	
• Yearn	• Yield	• Young		
• Zeal	• Zest	• Zip		

Intellectual or Mental Influences

The mind is the generator of thoughts. Thoughts are things—they can do harm or good.

║ "My tormentor is myself left over from yesterday." Deepak Chopra ║

Kinds of Intellectual and Mental Influences

Column 1	Column 2
• Abuse or neglect of intellectual or mental health	• Chemical imbalance—internal source, external source
• Environmental imbalance	• Immune system disturbance
• Inherited/genetic imbalance or disease	• Intellectual/mental imbalance or disturbance (schizophrenia, multiple personality disorder)
• Mental attitude	• Mental
• Psychological	• Stress
• Task	

Thought Patterns or Thought Habits

Column 1	Column 1
• Thoughts from: self or others	• Hurried decisions
• Thoughts to: self or others	• Incorrect assessment of situations
• Thoughts: positive (+) negative (-) neutral ( )	• Under/overenthusiastic
• Thoughts: too many or not enough	• Flares up
• Thoughts: harmful or helpful	• No perseverance
• Thoughts: worthy or unworthy	• Too much self importance
• Day dreaming: too much/not enough focused/ unfocused	• Lack of energy
• Deep thinking or shallow thinking	• Avoids difficult decisions
• Past life carried over: need to let go thoughts or thought patterns	• Lack of initiative
• The <u>four</u> most damaging self images: Fear image, Inferiority image, Inadequate image, Dependency image	• Task

Personal Philosophy

Column 1	Column 2
• Anarchy	• Deceitful
• Democracy	• Fantasy
• Optimism	• Pessimism
• Reality	• Relativism
• Skeptical	• Spiritual
• Truthful	

(continued)

Intellectual or Mental Influences, continued

Clues about Intellectual and Mental Influences

- Consider the level or type of intelligence rather than judging a person as being less than you. This is a list of **Gardner's Seven Intelligences:**
  - – Visual/Spatial Intelligence
  - – Logical/Mathematical Intelligence
  - – Verbal/Linguistic Intelligence
  - – Musical/Rhythmic Intelligence
  - – Bodily/Kinesthetic Intelligence
  - – Interpersonal/Social Intelligence
  - – Intrapersonal/Social Intelligence

- Whatever you put out into the Universe (to God), through emotion and intellectual action, the Universe reflects back.

> You are what your deep, driving desire is.
> As your desire is, so is your will.
> As your will is, so is your deed.
> As your deed is, so is your destiny.
>
> *Brahadaranyaka Upanishad*

Resolutions for Intellectual and Mental Influences

- Requires time to learn about:
  - – Emotional education
  - – Mental education
  - – Nutritional education
  - – Religious education
  - – Spiritual education
  - – Physical education
  - – Other study or exploration (see *Educational Issues* p. 87)

- Needs one or more of the following:
  - – Change one's thoughts.
  - – Allow a daily thought/ meditation time period.
  - – Nurture mental/ intellectual aspect of self.
  - – Keep thought patterns in line (focused).
  - – Modify a belief system (one's moral or ethical values)

- Therapists to consider:
  - – Counselor
  - – Hypnotist
  - – Mental hospital or facility
  - – Psychiatrist
  - – Psychologist
  - – Regression

- Goal setting:
  - – What is holding you back from achieving?
  - – Effort—lack of or too much
  - – A sense of want combined with effort = success
  - – Want without effort = no success
  - – Self discovery

INFLUENCES ON SPIRIT ISSUES

Table of Contents

Energy Field Influences

There are a variety of definitions and approaches to dealing with or describing the energy fields around and within the human system:

- Subtle body
- Aura
- Meridians
- Chakras

Subtle Body

One definition of the energy field is the subtle body (the nonphysical psychic body) that is superimposed on our physical bodies. It contains the more spiritual parts of ourselves. It is measured as an electromagnetic force field. (Kirlian photography has produced photographic images of it.) The aura is the external manifestation of the subtle body. The chakras, discussed later, are manifestations of the subtle body at the core of the physical body.

Aura

The aura is often referred to as a force field of energy surrounding the soul and lower bodies on which impressions, thoughts, feelings, words, and actions of the individual and other individuals are registered. Some scientists have referred to this as the L-field which they feel controls the manifestations of the physical body.

The aura is continually vibrating and changing size and shape. People also note a variety of colors flowing around and within the aura. Different colors and their locations denote different goings on or aspects of the person, their health, mental balance, consciousness, etc. Many people have the ability to see the energy field around the body. In fact, all people can do so if they relax, slightly blur their eyes and not get too tense in their focus.

Integrity of the aura can affect the body. If the aura is imbalanced, the body may be left open to illness. Energy may be transferred from one person's aura to another's (intentionally/unintentionally). By visualization and auric exercises one may enhance and strengthen one's aura.

Layers of the Aura

There are different descriptions and definitions of the layers of the aura. We chose the following explanation to differentiate between different levels and layers to assist in your understanding of the aspects of the aura. We are in no way saying this is the one and only way to describe the aura.

Laverne E. Denyer describes the aura as a set of 11 layers, calling them the Energetic Bodies. To be more precise, these layers are actually overlapping and interrelated energy patterns that share the same space.

For the purpose of this *To Our Health* Workbook, we group Denyer's 11 layers into layers B, C, D and E. This Workbook uses Denyer's system to help locate issues and problems because many of them may not be directly at the physical level, but may lie on one of the layers of the aura.

The Physical Body (layer A in the *Body Chart* p. 17)	
The Material Base Aspect (layer B in the *Body Chart*)	The Material Base Aspect consists of four layers described by Denyer: Physical Body, Etheric Body, Emotional Body, and Mental Body. These provide a solid base for the soul to partner within the material world. (They embody the masculine aspect of the energy bodies—the force that enables life). This is the portion of humanity which is born, lives and dies. It has finite existence and is tied to the earth's laws. Here lie desire, hope, fear and limitation. It fears death as it is a real ending for this level of being.
The Fulcrum Aspect (layer C in the *Body Chart*)	The Fulcrum Aspect consists of a single layer—the Astral Body, which is a transition linkage between spirit and matter. When this aspect is well, there is a balance between esoteric (spiritual) and temporal (earthly). This manifests as a practical, prosperous person with wisdom and connection to higher powers. It has an androgynous aspect that allows force and creativity to blend in harmony.
The Individual Soul Aspect of the Aura (layer D in the *Body Chart*)	This layer carries an individual's soul connection. Spirit becomes manifest as a conscious being. It gives separation from the God Force Aspect. The soul in this aspect is eternal and knows and remembers the connection with the God Force. There is no death of the soul. The Individual Soul Aspect consists of four layers—Etheric Template Body, Celestial Body, Ketheric Template Body, and the Auric Body. They embody the feminine aspect of the energetic bodies, the creative energy that defines and directs. These layers provide a foundation for the spirit to manifest as material. These layers also nourish and support the Material Aspect in daily survival and growth.
The God Force Aspect of the Aura (layer E in the *Body Chart*)	God Force Aspect originated from one source and will eventually reunite with the ONE CONSCIOUSNESS. It has no gender classification (all and none). It is our connection with the primal creative force. Our oversoul and our other lives reside here. It manifests as pure spiritual energy beyond the earthly plane. The God Force Aspect consists of three layers—First and Second Cosmic Bodies and God/Tao Body. These layers are universal, relating to all energies from the universe and other dimensions. (The layers A through D are connected to the earthly plane.)
The Higher Soul Self (layer F in the *Body Chart*)	When we come out of our mother's womb and become earthly beings then we get surrounded by our Higher **Soul** Self, which represents the outer layer of our energy field.

Layers B through E above summarize Denyer's description of the various levels of the aura or energy field. Our *Body Chart* on p. 17 includes outlines of the above discussed layers. Issues and problems may have their source or origin from aspects beyond the physical plane as well as on the physical plane.

Aura Colors

Listed below are colors that may be found in the aura. Varying shades, muddiness, clarity, and other aspects of the colors imply different states. The *Emotional Gauge for HHH Dowsing* on p. 57 lists the colors and chakra associated with a color.

Aura Colors

Red	Symbol of life, strength, vitality, strong mind. Virile, materialistic, passionate, hatred, revenge.
Orange	Health, vitality. Vital force. Soul of energy. Live wire. Domination of others through force of vital qualities. Positions of responsibility. Easier to rule than to serve. Usually well balanced. It is expressive of wisdom and reasoning powers.
Yellow	God Aspect. Golden signifies soul qualities. Astral mental forces. Symbolizes thought and mental concentration. Light and presence of intellect. Bright, optimistic, intelligent, and capable (business). High-spirited. (A grayish-yellow color typically signifies fear.)
Green	Individualism, regeneration, energy, and supply. Keynote of ego. Growth. Tendency towards prosperity and success. Multiplicity of ideas. Animated, versatile, thoughtful, adaptable. Freedom from bondage, independence, new life. (Pale green signifies healing power. Grayish green signifies pessimism, envy.)
Blue	Heaven's hue. Inspiration. Color of fortune. An artistic, harmonious nature and spiritual understanding. (Bright blue signifies self-reliance, confidence, loyalty, and sincerity. Poised, calm, spiritually aware. Cool and aloof. Tendency towards teaching, singing, or lecturing.) (Grayish blue signifies melancholy. Ice blue signifies an intellectual tendency.)
Indigo	Very high spiritual vibrations. High intuition. Ability to meditate deeply. Follows inner guidance in making decisions and finding solutions. Dedication to high ideals. Worshipful sense. Expansion of inner vision and awareness.
Violet/ purple	Extremely high vibrations. Appeals to more sensitive and soul conscious people rather than masses. Path of service and dedication to highest ideals. Combines spirituality of blue with addition of red elements of vitality and power. Color of the Initiate and Adept. Ray of power and influence. True greatness and worthiness. Disinterested love and wisdom. (Orchid color signifies idealism.)
Pink	Mystic color. Quiet, refined, modest. Fond of beauty and artistic surroundings. Great and lasting devotion.
Brown	Capacity for organization and orderly management. Industry and diligent work. Ruling color of convention. Starting point of ambition and power. Material and commercial. Painstaking perseverance. Earthy. (Dull brown signifies low energy.)
Gray	Fear, boredom, repressed anger, initiation.
Black	Depression, protection.
White	Highly spiritual (rarely seen)
Gold/ silver	Pure knowing and intuition. Very developed psychically.
Trans- parent	Reader, restorer, loved, void, truth, pure light.
Clear	Endurance, here—in the now, clear decision-maker, uses divine blue print, mystic.

Problems of the Aura/Influences of the Aura on Mind Issues

1	There can be malfunctions of magnetic field or electro-biochemical field.
2	There can be holes, gaps, balloons or other enlargements of areas on aura

Resolutions for Aura Problems or Influences

- Need to balance auric field because it is overextended or underdeveloped.
- Need to work with:

– Animals	– Belief systems	– Chakras	– Colors	– Energy movement
– Gem stones	– Healers	– Mantra	– Meditation	– Numbers
– People	– Positive thought	– Sound	– Symbols	

Chi Energy and Meridians

There are numerous energy flows, lines, vortices, and centers in and around the body. Awareness of these areas helps one tune into problems or issues. There may be a blockage or energy flow problem that needs to be addressed and treated to encourage better health.

Chi or Qi is a Chinese word for a concept of energy that is found throughout the universe. It is in both organic and inorganic material. It is a form of vital energy verging on being both matter and energy. The proper flow or balance of this energy in the body is important for the body to be in health.

Meridians are pathways for the flow of chi energy. They are found on and in the human body and have been measured electronically, thematically, and radioactively. Acupressure and acupuncture points are found along these meridians. (The science of acupuncture has been a part of Chinese culture and civilization for thousands of years.) There are 14 major meridians that interconnect the various body organs and parts.

These meridians are associated with life functions of body organs. They carry communication between parts of the body. They flow either up or down the body. Their flow is on the surface, but they interconnect within the torso. There is no beginning or end to the flow; the energy flows from one meridian to another like a wheel would continuously roll across a surface. Meridians have both positive and negative energy charges.

When energy flow is unrestricted, the body harmonizes the flow to keep it functioning well. Stress and other problems may hamper the flow (overloading the circuits).

Pressure on, massaging or passing hands over the meridians may help stabilize the flow. For more information about meridians and ways to use them to bring about better health, consult the *Touch for Health Workbook*.

Chakras

The concept of chakras has been found in cultures and in many belief systems in India for thousands of years. The chakras are described as vortices through which energy flows both in and out of the body. The power or energy that is involved with the chakras comes from Kundalini or evolutionary energy and from a spiritual force within. Chakras are to be found on all layers and levels (spiritual, physical, mental, emotional, auric, etc.).

There are seven main chakras, shown on the front-facing figure in the *Body Chart* p. 17 and listed in the *Emotional Gauge for HHH Dowsing* p. 57. There are more than 100 chakras that can be located all over the body.

A person's development affects which chakras are predominantly used. Some people have too much energy located in the lower chakras, leaving the central and upper chakras weak. Other people overemphasize the upper chakras, leaving the lower chakras weak. Chakras need to have balanced energy flows. Neglect of one aspect of the self does not bring about balance or harmony, but produces an imbalance that might open one to a variety of problems.

Use your dowsing tool with the chakras and aura layers in the *Body Chart* on p. 17 if you need to locate problem areas.

Locations of the Seven Main Chakra Centers

The seven chakra centers listed below are also listed on the *Body Chart*, because we often find people with chakra imbalances when doing dowsing work.

Root chakra	Focus: Physical. Life force. Color: Red. Glands: Adrenals. Musical note: C
Sex chakra	Focus: Emotional creativity, physical creativity. Color: Red-orange. Glands: Ovaries, prostate, testicles. Musical note: D
Solar Plexus chakra	Focus: Mental/emotional personal power. Color: Yellow. Gland: Spleen. Musical note: E
Heart chakra	Focus: Mental/spiritual healing, feelings. Color: Green. Gland: Thymus. Musical note: F
Throat chakra	Focus: Mental/spiritual healing, communication, power and creative energy. Color: Sky blue Glands: Thyroid, parathyroid. Musical note: G
Third Eye chakra	Focus: Spiritual visualization, cosmic consciousness, intuition, healing. Color: Indigo. Gland: Pituitary. Musical note: A
Crown chakra	Focus: Spiritual wisdom, integration, cosmic consciousness. Color: Electric ultraviolet, iridescent, mother-of-pearl, rainbow, white. Gland: Pineal. Musical note: B

A great deal of information is becoming available regarding chakras, their clearing, unblocking, opening and developing. Interaction with people has a great effect on one's chakras. Some people will unconsciously pull energy from open or unguarded chakras. When we interact with others or are merely in their presence, chakras will react to them.

Awareness of this will be helpful in understanding why one might feel drained, invigorated, uncomfortable, and so forth around particular people. Often it is helpful to focus on, wear, hold or use colors that are associated with the various chakras to enhance or help. It has been noted that humming or singing some of the above mentioned musical notes will also help clear or stimulate the various chakras. Again we suggest you consult reading material or specialists if you need more information or help with chakras.

Problems with Chakras or Meridians
- Closed
- Too open
- Unbalanced
- Improper energy flow
- Not enough energy

Resolutions for Chakra or Meridian Problems
- Learn to: work with, manipulate, see, focus on.
- Work with elements: Earth, Water, Fire, Wood, Metal, Air.
- Use: visualization, energy: affirmations.
- Need to: heal, be energized, seal, let go.

Belief System (Religious) Influences

Below are listed a number of religious or belief systems that have been used by humanity and that can influence mind issues. This list is by no means complete.

- Christian-based beliefs
    - Adventist (Seventh Day; Church of God)
    - Church of Jesus Christ of Latter Day Saints (Mormons)
    - Friends (Quaker)
    - Lutheran
    - Mysticism (Christian)
    - Pentecostal (Assembly of God, Four Square)
    - Baptist (27 groups)
    - Eastern Orthodox
    - Greek Orthodox
    - Mennonite (similar to Amish)
    - Nazarene
    - Roman Catholic
    - Universalist
    - Church of Christ Scientist (Christian Science)
    - Episcopal (Anglican)
    - Jehovah's Witness
    - Methodist
    - Orthodox Presbyterian
    - Russian Orthodox
    - Unitarian
    - Satanism (Belief in God, Christ but focuses on evil/opposite of God)

- Animism
  It is the modern belief in forces of nature, and was the focus of the ancient ("dead") religions: Greek, Etruscan, Sumerian, etc.

- Buddhism
    - Buddhist Churches of America
    - Therevadan Buddhism (Burma, Ceylon)
    - Zen Buddhism (Japanese)
    - Chinese Buddhism
    - Tibetan Buddhism

- Confucianism (Chinese)
- Hinduism (India)
  Thousands of varieties of worship: Yoga, Gods/Goddesses, etc.

- Islam
    - Muslim/Moslem
    - Black Muslim
    - Sufi (Mystical Islam)

- Judaism (Orthodox, Conservative, Reformed, etc.)
- Native American religions

(continued)

Belief System (Religious) Influences, continued

- New Age
  New Age is a term for "modern" spiritual outlook. It incorporates beliefs in multiple areas—auras, chakras, energy vortexes, and powers and properties of plants or minerals, etc. One's practice may include all or only a few aspects. It focuses on recognition of one's own innate abilities with the assistance of other forces.

- Rastafarianism
- Self-directed (Eclectic)
  Consult encyclopedias and other references for religions and religious materials.

- Shamanism
- Spiritualism
  It may incorporate a variety of religious outlooks with many aspects. It looks at the power of Higher Force and its manifestations in the world around you.

- Taoism (Chinese)
- Shintoism (Japanese)
- Voodoo
  It is an ancient African-based belief system.

- Wiccan/Paganism
  It focuses on natural forces and a person's ability to make use of them

Problems or Issues Related to Religions/Belief Systems

1	Belief system is too limiting, structured, rigid.
2	Belief system lacks structure.
3	Belief system gives inadequate support.

Resolutions for Religions/Belief Systems

- Need to:
  Find a new system.
  Stay with an existing belief system.
  Work within religious system to develop self.
  Focus on working with others' self development.
- Become: missionary, teacher, lay person, disciple, volunteer.
- Belief/religious system is harmful / is helpful.
- Need to devote more/less: time, effort, money.
- Create: book, poetry, music, artwork, dance, ritual.
- Sing hymns.
- Meditate
- Religion/belief system: conscious, subconscious.

- Find belief system that:
  Focuses on social interaction.
  Focuses on personal development.
  Balances social/individual aspects.

- Should consider: becoming part of clergy, leaving clergy.
- Rely on own intuition in regards to beliefs.
- Read more/read less religious material.
- Problems with: fellow members, religious hierarchy, clergy.
- Pray.
- Preach.

Karmic Influences

Also see *Soul Levels* p. 84.

> As above, so below.
> Whatever ye sow--so shall ye reap.
> For every action, there is a reaction.
> Voids must be filled.
> All things change.
> Give to receive.
> Polarities will seek balance.

In Sanskrit, karma means "reaction follows action"—what you send out, you get back. Karma is neither good nor bad. It may be painful, but it promotes growth. From lifetime to lifetime, man determines his fate by his action, including thoughts, feelings, words, and deeds.

(Much of the following material on karma comes from <u>Kundalini and the Chakras</u> by Genevieve Lewis Paulson.)

Ego attachments are one source of karma or are apt to create it. One needs to develop an attitude of detachment. (This does not mean non-caring. One may actually care more deeply and risk more when detached.)

An "eye for an eye" concept does not help let go karma. Rather, the concept and use of forgiveness helps to let go karma. One might also let go karma by understanding what one does, feels, or thinks. It is also helpful to ask a Higher Force to help you with letting go.

After letting go karma, one must change, or else end up drawing the same or similar situation back—often worse than before. In order to grow, we must all go through learning experiences. It is our attitude and feelings towards these lessons and experiences that makes the difference in how we travel through our lives. Often our experiences are not the result of karma but are opportunities that are being presented to us. We must be aware that new energies are encountered during our growth or evolution as spiritual beings. Often opportunities give one the sense of being pushed towards the situation, while karmic situations often give the sense of one being pulled towards the action.

Personal Karma

Situational—Anything you have done to someone else in a past life is returned in kind to you by that person in this life. (This cycle may go on for several lifetimes.)

Attitudinal—Example: all past life anger toward life or others affects all you do in this life. (This karma attracts similar attitudes and feelings that you send out.) Be aware of unhealthy attitudes, and let them go. For example, it is best to fill yourself with love.

Karma of Others

People often get caught up in other people's karma. Worrying or interfering when we shouldn't are causes of this entanglement. Rather than worry, send blessings. At times it is good to help and assist others. However, before doing so use prayer, intuition, and consideration to see if it is in the best interest of all to get involved.

Group Karma

A group can develop karma that needs to be worked on as individuals or as the group that initiated the karma. Be aware and conscious of your group and its actions; don't create unwanted or unnecessary karma.

Conscious Choice of Karma

Prior to coming into this life people make a choice as to what and how much karma they wish to let go or develop so that their growth process may be enhanced. For example, some people may choose to develop an illness and then exceed the limitations supposedly placed upon them by that illness. Again remember that we play a strong role in choosing our lives and what occurs during them.

Karmic Record

This record is said to be written in the book of Life (in Akasha) and in the etheric body. This is a record of the individual's use of energy since the descent of the soul into matter. It is a record of cause-effect sequences made by the soul's interaction with other souls.

Possible Sources of Karmic Influences

1	Creating karma	Law of Cause and Effect and Retribution
2	Energy in action	Unfinished business -- in this life-- in past life
3	Karmic residue	Time karma
4	Karma associated with: empires, civilizations, countries, states, provinces, city, town, village, estate (for clues, check a world history atlas, and check through time periods)	
5	Karma associated with continents: Asia, Africa, Europe, North America, South America, Australia, Antarctica	
6	Family karma	Other's karma
7	Group karma	Race karma
8	Personal karma: situational	Personal karma: attitudinal

Resolution of Karmic Influences

- Receive, to balance.   Give, to balance.
- Change an attitude.
- Focus on karma.   Do not focus on karma.
- Regression: is helpful, is not helpful.

Possessive Forces, Entities, Attachments, and Afflictions

Often sensitive people will feel a presence or a change in the air around them. More often than not a simple request that the being/entity leave and seek the White Light is all that is needed. Many times a presence may also be that of a relative or loved one that feels as though certain issues have not been resolved, or certain life tasks have not been completed.

Cautions about Attracting Unwanted Forces

People full of Light energy attract many dark pockets within entities who are searching for Light. People who are consciously on the path need to have constant awareness and protection to guard for and help these entities to move on to the Divine Light (not with malice, but with kind intent and love). If an entity is not ready to be helped, respect that; later, when the entity is ready, you can help it.

Thoughts of jealousy, hate, destruction, envy, and fear invite and attract these same feelings which are part of many incarnate and unicarnate beings. It is in one's best interest to avoid and refrain from indulging in these emotions or one will risk encounters and attachments.

Drugs, alcohol, and other harmful substances to the body, mind, and spirit also tend to weaken and leave people open to these forces.

If you are in the habit of collecting artifacts, antiques, stones, crystals, or if you have stored or been given a dead animal such as a bird, an insect, or road kill, be aware that these items might be anchoring points for beings (human and nonhuman).

Be aware of beings (sometimes people) who want to get control of your mind, soul, or being. They use any means that are at their disposal. Be aware of the use of electronic, chemical, hypnotic, or sexual methods. Often they may try to reach and/or influence you on the feeling or emotional level. Psychic "hooks" may also be place upon you. These are used to reel in, pull on you, distract you, and may often cause a sense of physical pain or discomfort. Awareness and protection using the White Light are often your best defense.

See *Resolutions* and *Prayers to Remove the Attachment* on p. 81 for antidotes.

Purpose and Types of Possessive Forces, Entities, and Attachments

- **Is the purpose of the force:** Positive   Negative   Helpful   Neutral   Harmful

Column 1	Column 2	Column 3
• Atlantean entities	• Automatic writing	• Black magic entities
• Body bound entities	• Crawl-in (see Note 1)	• Curse put on you or on family from this lifetime or past life time
• Dark forces	• Disembodied soul entity	• Earthbound entities
• Emotional entities	• Fear entities	• Gargoyles
• Gloom, doom, and disaster	• Goblins	• Gray entities
• Gremlins	• Haunted house	• Hospital (any place you go has vibrations)
• Lemurian entities	• Mass consciousness (a curse from another dimension)	• Negative spirit attachments
• Ouija board	• Past life entities	• Poltergeist
• Residue haunting (residual haunting)	• Satanic entities	• Scared soul entity
• Spell	• Spirit possession of the soul	• Voodoo spell
• Walk-in (see Note 2 below)	• Witchcraft spell	

Note 1: A **crawl-in** is a soul that enters a mother's womb. This soul has been weakened by past experience and requires special care. It may be born with karmic ties and physical defects necessary for its growth and development and also for the growth and development of the people it encounters.

Note 2: **Walk-in**: Some souls choose to leave the earthly plane. In some cases, when the soul leaves, another may take its place. This is known as a "walk-in" soul. Often these souls are intent on helping with world enlightenment.

Possible Effects or Afflictions Resulting from Attachments

1	Sudden changes in behavior: eating, drinking, or sleeping.
2	Increased negative emotions: Depression, increase in anger, rebelliousness, fear, panic, suicidal tendencies.
3	Physical pain, with usually no lab or x-ray findings. Pain does not respond to traditional medical treatment.
4	Serious illness (unknown cause): Persistent, non-responsive infections possibly caused by attached earthbound entities who suffered from or died of infection. (When entity leaves, the infection leaves.) Unusual inflammatory or metabolic disorders and blood dyscrasias.
5	Loss of energy: sudden decrease of physical energy.
6	Sudden onset of alcohol or drug abuse: Possessing entity is usually one who indulged in drugs or alcohol. When the entity leaves so does urge for alcohol and drugs.
7	Memory and concentration problems: One who is accustomed to easy learning and high grades abruptly changes to low performance and poor grades.
8	Inner voices: Voices express reaction or point of view which differs from one's normal perspective.
9	Multiple personality disorder: Multiples are often caused by entities. Careful evaluation is necessary.
10	Repetitious nightmares: Dreams contain elements of violence or of struggle against threatening forces.

Resolutions to Remove the Attachment

Be aware that all thoughts and feelings are not necessarily your own. Surround yourself, family, friends, places, cities, and ultimately everything with the Light of Love as protection.

Recommended remedies are a bath, salt, and/or aromatherapy.

Burn sage in the house, and waft the smoke over yourself. Or burn incense.

Wear silk.

Prayers to Remove the Attachment

Below are some prayers that might be used when faced with issues described on preceding pages. It is suggested that if one feels uncomfortable or troubled one might consider consulting a professional.

Forgiveness Prayer

Thank you, Father, for everything that has happened to me, whether it was painful or pleasurable. I am praying to give and ask for forgiveness. Thank you (*name*) for doing to me all that you have done. Forgive me (*name*) for doing all that I have done to you.

Prayers to Clear Entities

Dear Lord,
Please bless this eternal being so that it is cleared, on the physical, mental, emotional, and spiritual level, of all possessive forces, entities, attachments, and afflictions. I ask that before they leave they heal the aura of attachment, and I ask that they get guided to the Light and surrounded by unconditional love. I let you go, and you are free.
Thank you, God. Bless Love, Bless Love, Bless Love.

— ✑ —

For all those who are lost and wandering, we ask they receive guidance to the Light. Are you ready to go to the Light? (If the answer is yes, you may say a short prayer to help them to move on.)
Thank you, God.

— ✑ —

Please bless this house so it is clean of entities. I ask that they receive guidance to the Light. I let you go. Bless you. May your spirit be at peace. You are free.
Thank you, God.

Request to Leave

If you are not in or of the White or Gold Light, Please leave!
Bless Love.

Psychic Senses and Other Resources

The realization of psychic or extrasensory abilities is not something that is necessarily magical or mystical. Rather, one might consider these as some of the unused abilities that are part of every normal human. They are merely awaiting discovery and use.

In many ways we are only partly alive and aware. We have developed certain patterns of perceiving, thinking, and imagining. While these are highly functional, they tend to limit our more expansive abilities, visions, and thoughts. Just as we limit our muscles and flexibility by becoming rigid and armored in our movement, we have limited our mental powers by covering them with fears, intellectual conflicts, and contradicting belief systems.

Psychic healing is the best and highest form of healing known to man. But even psychic healing will not and cannot effect a permanent cure unless a client changes habits of living and lives in accordance with nature's laws.

Listed below are a number of abilities noted in people throughout human existence. These may also be referred to as extrasensory perception or intuition. Read with an open mind and begin to recognize these as yours.

Psychic Senses

Automatic writing	Writing with the aid of a spiritual guide or teacher. Often one is not conscious of what is being written.
Channeling	Ability to receive direction or information from the higher self and universe. Information comes from a source other than the ego.
Clairaudience	The ability to hear a spirit within or without one's mind.
Clairsentience	The ability to send and receive thought between spirit and self (comparable to telepathy, inner voice in mind).
Clairvoyance	The ability to perceive situations and information at a distance directly, without the mediation of another mind or vehicle.
Precognition	Future access. The ability to perceive information across time and into the future.
Psychokinesis/ Telekinesis	The ability to influence the nature of physical matter without any physical contact, purely with the power of the mind.
Psychometry	The ability to touch something and sense its relationship to people, time, etc. entirely through contact with the object. (It involves sensing of the object's energy field and the imprints left upon it.)
Retrocognition	Past access. The ability to perceive previous events and information back through time.
Telepathy	The ability to communicate with another mind without the use of any of the basic five senses.
Vibration empathy	The ability to accomplish such sensory activities as divining, reading auras, astral traveling, healing, and locating lost objects.

Tools and Teachers

Column 1	Column 2	Column 3
• Ancient arts, beliefs, abilities	• Animal totems	• Aromatherapy
• Astrology	• Crystals	• Dowsing
• Drumming	• Fetishes	• Guru or other teacher
• Healing: psychic, spiritual	• Herbs	• Medicine man/woman
• Numerology	• Out of body (astral projection)	• Palmistry
• Past life regression	• Phrenology	• Psychic surgery
• Quantum physics	• Quest (women)	• Ritual tools
• Rituals or other ceremonies	• Seeing or scrying	• Shaman
• Smoking, smudging, incense	• Subtle body awareness	• Sweat lodge
• Symbology	• Talismans	• Tarot or other card reading
• Trance work	• UFO's	• Vision Quest (men)

Guides and Guardians

Many psychics state that we are always surrounded by many spiritual beings of whom we are not aware. We have little or no awareness of the many levels and planes. Often, we only need to ask for assistance or guidance and this will be provided in one form or another. What is best for our growth and development may not necessarily be something that we enjoy, but rather might be something painful and uncomfortable. We must be open to all our experiences and find what is meant for us to see or grow from with this lesson.

Spiritual guide	This is often a guardian that works with you prior to your coming to the earth plane. Their purpose is usually karma-influenced, and it can be twofold: • Clear karma owed to you • See that you fulfill your chosen path The guardian is usually opposite in gender, for they can add the love or strength needed. They know what they need to do and work hard to see completion. Trust in and knowledge of them may help one through this life's journey.
Provider guide	This guide is assigned to work with you, to bring what you need and give direction. They often work weeks ahead of you. The main work occurs when one strays off the path. They then need to provide a way back to your path. Faith and trust best ways to receive assistance from these guides. They usually choose to help the person.
Personal guide	This guide is usually a family member, friend or teacher who wishes to help from the spirit world.
Angels, members of the Brotherhood of Light, etc.	Many religions and belief systems throughout the world have mentioned angels and gods. Often these are higher evolved beings that are involved in the evolutionary growth process of all beings. They are often nearby to assist, observe or instruct.

Soul Influences

For other clues, see the *Table of Contents* p. 68 for *Influences on Spiritual Issues*.

The soul remembers that the soul is that which you are at every given moment of life.

> Every soul is a portion of God. Each one of us is a soul, a portion of the
> Divine Energy that brought us into being. We stand in relationship to God,
> or the Creative Energy of the universe, as a sunbeam to the sun, or a drop of
> water to the ocean. We stand in relation to our body as a man to his house or
> his garment. You don't go to heaven, you grow to heaven.
> Edgar Cayce

Each soul has chosen, or has been chosen, to enter this life to complete a lesson or assist in lessons for growth in the completion of this earthly cycle. There are many levels above and below this earthly cycle. Each level requires the soul reach a certain attainment of knowledge and wisdom before it may go on to the next. There are many levels of evolution for the soul. Reincarnation may occur many times prior to the soul's achieving another level. Souls may also advance levels in a single lifetime. There are also several different types of souls, each with different characteristics, goals and emphases throughout their lifetimes. To explore this aspect further, read Messages from Michael by Chelsea Yarbro.

Ages of Consciousness

This concerns development of souls throughout earth's history. The majority of souls go through stages mentioned below for *Soul Levels*. At present we are at the verge of reaching a majority of Old Souls in the earth cycle. To encourage soul development, be conscious of and incorporate laws of universal consciousness into your life.

The Laws of Universal Consciousness

1. Unconditional love for all creation	2. Honest feelings and knowing them	3. Non-interference
4. Realization of cause and effect	5. Natural order	6. Patience
7. Responsibility	8. Progression	9. Oneness
10. Forgiveness	11. Serving	12. Detachment/surrender

Soul Levels

Before asking about and dowsing for issues related to soul level, ask for permission, as described on p. 23, on all levels of client's and your consciousness.

When dealing with other people it may be worth one's while to **check on the soul level** that any particular person is working from. If you are dealing with an Infant or Baby soul, and at times a Young Soul, you may find it difficult to communicate or convince them of certain points of view. At this time it is not worth your while to become frustrated or upset with these people. Accept and bless them for the stage of growth that they are presently in. Many people become stuck on certain levels because they have not completed certain lessons of letting go and accepting, and consequently remain stuck in their present

Soul Influences and **Soul Levels,** continued

life. Again, ultimately the person chooses when to grow. There can be no forced growth or change from the outside.

Before Earthly Soul Cycle—Plants, Animals, Mineral Kingdom

- **Unborn Soul** One who is waiting to incarnate into earthly life. A fragment that has little sense of self-awareness. May yet be closely tied to Divine Energy, or has been separated for a great length of time. Very little influence on others. Many are just waiting to rejoin soul groups.

Earthly Soul Cycles

- **Infant Soul** (Firstborn) Born to simple surroundings. Fearful of new experiences. Does not know difference between right and wrong.
- **Baby Soul** Focus on preservation of status quo. Highly conservative.
- **Young Soul** Sets impossible goals (idealistic, materialistic). High sense of ego. Wants success, acceptance.
- **Mature Soul** Seeker of higher knowledge. Open to psychic experience and abilities. An Old Soul is trying to emerge.
- **Old Soul** Not materialistic. Tends to focus on the service of others. Tends towards individualism, but not forceful as with younger souls.

Beyond Earthly Soul Cycles

- **Transcendental Soul** Very high soul. Incarnates for specific purpose. Prepares way for the "Infinite Soul." Development beyond earthly soul cycles.
- **Infinite Soul** Comes to earth to change mankind's course. In touch or harmony with Divine Consciousness

During work on this book, Anneliese and Doris recognized situations where soul levels existed in addition to levels listed above. We will address this at a future time.

Sources of and Resolutions for Soul Problems

‖ You can't save another soul, if you are going to lose your own in the process. ‖

- Soul fragmentation: disruption of the soul due to trauma, violation, shock, etc.
- Parts of the soul have dispersed and need to be retrieved and joined back to the whole.
- Is there a veil over the soul?
- Is the soul blocked, depleted, subdued, chained, discarded, trapped, split?
- Is a supernatural force in there?
- Some souls are and feel off-zapped, knotted, tortured, outspoken, escaping, squashed, snipped, beggars, shattered, kinked, rebellious, entangled, living in a pattern, bonded with other souls, duality habit.
- Is the Soul a mate, seeker, twin, twin flame, walk-in (see p. 80), crawl-in (see p. 80)?
- The soul needs to be elevated to a higher consciousness.
- The soul needs cleansing, needs to be heard, needs to be freed.
- The soul is lost—seek guidance and help from higher sources to enable soul to find the Light.
- **Pray.**
- **Bless Love.**

INFLUENCES ON BODY-MIND-SPIRIT ISSUES

Table of Contents

Educational Issues and Resolutions

See also *Nutritional Influences* p. 51, *Physical Influences* p. 54, *Negative Emotional Influences* p. 58, *Intellectual or Mental Influences* p. 66, and *Sexual Issues* p. 94. Also check for books, leaflets, etc. for material pertaining to educational issues.

Kind of School that's Related to an Educational Issue

Column 1	Column 2	Column 3
• Day care or child care	• Preschool	• Head Start
• Kindergarten	• Grade school	• High school
• College	• University	• Technical school
• Vocational school	• Graduate school	• Medical school
• Law school	• Public school	• Parochial school
• Babysitter or other sitter		

Learning Disabilities and other Difficulties that Affect Learning

Column 1	Column 2	Column 3
• ADHD (ADD HD combined)	• Attention Deficit Disorder (ADD)	• At risk
• Autism	• Cognitively disabled	• Drug or alcohol-related problems
• Dysgraphia	• Dyslexia	• Dysphasia
• Educational, social, or authority fears	• Hyperactivity Disorder (HD)	• Slow learner
• Stuttering	• Visual, auditory, and/or speech difficulties	

Behavioral Issues, Overview

Items listed below might be areas of problems and concerns.

Column 1	Column 2	Column 3
• Accident prone	• Allergies	• Bites nails
• Clumsy	• Conservative	• Constipated
• Daydreams	• Defiant/hard to discipline	• Difficulty budgeting time
• Difficulty concentrating	• Difficulty following directions	• Difficulty giving directions
• Difficulty making decisions	• Difficulty telling time	• Disturbing to others
• Does not handle stress	• Excitable	• Fidgety
• Fights	• Has nightmare	• Headaches
• Immature for age	• Impatient	• Impulsive
• Lacks confidence	• Leaves projects incomplete	• Letter or number reversals
• Lies	• Not enough school/too much school	• Moody
• Over active	• Poor eye/hand coordination	• Poor handwriting
• Poor reading comprehension	• Reckless	• Rests arm on head while writing
• Rubs eyes a lot	• Sensitive	• Slow in completing work
• Stops in middle of game	• Talks too much	• Teaser
• Unpopular	• Unpredictable	• Wets bed

(continued)

Educational Issues and Resolutions, continued

Resolutions and Tasks to Remedy Educational, Learning, and Behavioral Issues

1	Be careful of medications that are prescribed for some of these "disabilities". Medications may be more harmful than helpful. Discuss with physician carefully. Consider alternative approaches.
2	Need to leave school. Need to return to school.
3	Need to get a degree in high school or college or technical school.
4	Change classes or subject (minor major). Change job/ work place.
5	Education needed on the social, emotional, mental and spiritual plane. Formative preschool years.
6	Need for educational discipline, nurturing because of behavioral or emotional problems and difficulty (see the next page).
7	Check for visual, auditory and/or speech difficulties. Check for positive/negative affirmations.
8	Need to develop/accept responsibility. Check for child's readiness for school.
9	Need for references and resources. Attend or be part of PTO, PTA, school-sponsored activities (musical, sports, etc.).
10	Challenge yourself to try something new. Create a new idea.
11	Dance. Describe attitude toward authority.
12	Describe self as a servant. Express an emotion to fit a situation.
13	Feel thankful. Give a problem a new solution.
14	Imagine letting someone go to take care of him/herself. Laugh.
15	Make a choice. Memory.
16	Move in joy. Name encouraging words.
17	Offer choice of foods (sugar, fruit, etc.). Offer one item in exchange for another.
18	Organize some numbers or objects. Picture self in situation where could get public approval/disapproval.
19	Read. Relax—move freely.
20	See yourself in a new position in the future—job, family, etc.
21	Set long term and short term goal. Share a feeling about self with someone.
22	Sing; follow a tune. Sit perfectly still for 30 seconds.
23	Speak in a loving tone. Think about finishing a project.
24	Think about giving self and others the freedom to make mistakes.
25	Think about the future. Think of someone whose approval you need.
26	Visualize.
27	Write "the Past" on a piece of paper and have them let it go (burn it, bury it, tear it apart and throw it away, etc.).

Family Issues and Resolutions

For more clues, also see the following issues and resolutions: *Educational Issues* p. 87; *Financial Issues* p. 91; *Relationship Issues* p. 93; *Sexual Issues* p. 94; *Social Issues* p. 95. And consult *Emotional Gauge for HHH Dowsing* p. 57.

A person's spirit can say it's a family issue even if people involved aren't blood-related.

‖ Buried issues are still alive. ‖

Kind of Family Relationship

- Married
- Mother's side
- Separated

- Unmarried
- Father's side
- Divorced

- His side
- Living together
- Common-law

- Her side
- Living apart
- Cross religious marriage

- Interracial

- Non-traditional family:
  - lesbian
  - foster
  - gay
  - bigamy
  - single parent
  - polygamy
  - adopted
  - polyandry

Blood-related		Not Blood-related		
• Mother	• Nephew	• Husband/wife	• Step son/daughter	• Coworker
• Father	• Niece	• Ex-spouse	• Ex-step son/daughter	• Ex-coworker
• Brother	• Aunt	• Adopted parents	• Step brother/sister	• Professional
• Sister	• Uncle	• Adopted children	• Ex-step brother	• Boss
• Son	• Grandfather	• Lover	• Ex-step-sister	• Ex-boss
• Daughter	• Grandmother	• Ex-lover	• Daughter/son-in-law	• Godchild
• Twin	• Cousin	• Brother/sister-in-law	• Ex-daughter-in-law	• God parents
• Grandson	• Cousin 1st,2nd,3rd	• Ex-brother/ sister-in-law	• Ex-son-in-law	• Child care provider
• Grand-daughter	• Great grand-parent	• Stepfather/mother	• Boyfriend	
		• Ex-stepfather/mother	• Ex-boyfriend	• Baby-sitter
	• Great-great grandparent	• Father/mother-in-law	• Girlfriend	
		• Ex-father/mother-in-law	• Ex-girlfriend	• Clergy member
		• Step-grandparents	• Friend	
		• Ex-step-grandparents	• Neighbor	• Authority figure
		• Twin	• Ex-neighbor	
			• Spirit	• Teacher

Family Issues

- Abuse: emotional, physical, mental, sexual, spiritual, financial
- Clinging: bondage, jealousy, envy, unreturned love, obsessive love
- Possessiveness: towards others, from others
- Generations ago—issues or family history that is hidden or despised

- Aversion: hatred, anger
- Cultural / ethnic differences
- Religious differences
- Thought pollution from family

Resolutions for Family Issues

- Issues need to be resolved through you? or through your relative?

- This is not your issue, let it be.

Financial Issues and Resolutions

See also other influences on Body-Mind-Spirit: *Educational Issues*, *Family Issues*, and so forth.

Financial issues can be for oneself or for others.

Kind of Financial Issue

Column 1	Column 2
• Accountant financial planner: consult / change / need/ do not need	• Allowances for children
• Business: own/ should not own a business	• Business: sell it
• Child support	
• Estates, wills, inheritance	• Gains
• Gambling debt	• Gambling in a lottery
• Goal setting: required, modify, use, do not use	
• Health-related bills: hospital, doctor, prescriptions, tests, other	• House or building sale
• Insurance: life, disability, health, home, auto, disaster	
• Investment of money in stock market: buy, sell, avoid	• Investment of money: is it proper?
• Losses	
• Money owed to family or relative or friends	• Money owed to you from family or friends
• Money: not enough	• Money: too much
• Necessities (food, clothing, shelter)	
• Payments for car	• Payments for credit card
• Payments for house	• Payments for mortgage
• Payments for school: loans or tuition	• Payments to bank
• Payments: general loans	
• Pleasure, enjoyment	• Retirement pension: enough money, not enough money
• Spending too little	• Spending too much
• Taxes: sales, property, IRS (federal), state, Social Security (federal)	
• Tithing for a religious organization: should give, should avoid	• To be financially independent, secure
• Unemployment benefits	• Welfare (AFDC)
• Work: deserve a raise	• Work: bonuses

Resolutions and Tasks to Remedy Financial Issues

- I welcome financial abundance
- To accept freely
- To allow myself to receive as well as give
- To appreciate what is given to me
- To be a financial success
- To be a good steward
- To be a good steward of my goals
- To be financially secure
- To be in control of my spending
- To be materially secure
- To be worthy of my wages
- To choose large goals that coordinate
- To consume only what I need
- To expect good fortune
- To gain my resources in a way that benefits all
- To generously share my abundance
- To give equally
- To give freely to others in need
- To give full worth to whom I am in service
- To have a job that I enjoy
- To have goods when I need them
- To have sufficient goods to meet my needs
- To have sufficient money to meet my goals
- To have sufficient resources to meet my goals
- To have the necessities of life
- To make choices that cause financial increases
- To make wise investments
- To release poverty and welcome abundance
- To respect others property
- To save
- To share freely with God
- To share generously as I have ability
- To share with others in need
- To spend money wisely
- To succeed with money and goods
- To support myself well
- To use my resources in harmony with good
- To welcome abundance into my life
- To welcome wealth into my life

Relationship Issues and Resolutions

For more clues, also check other influences on Body-Mind-Spirit such as *Family Issues*, *Social Issues–Business*, etc.

Please note that this is a very limited list of possible people and problems.

Kind of Being in the Relationship

Column 1	Column 2
• Acquaintances	• Baby sitter or day care worker
• Boss	• Clergy or other religious occupation
• Coworker	• Customer
• Dentist	• Doctor
• Employee	• Employer
• Extraterrestrial/alien	• Family
• Farmer	• Female
• Health practitioner or other health field worker	• Law enforcement official
• Law-related: lawyer, judge, judicial employee	• Male
• Manager	• Neighbor
• Nurse	• Other occupations
• Partner	• Patient
• People	• Politician
• Real estate agent	• Social Worker
• Student	• Teacher
• Unknown	• Worker
• World	

Description of the Relationship Issue

1	A choice: of other(s), your choice
2	Envy: from/toward others
3	Feel responsible/do not feel responsible
4	His side/her side
5	Interpersonal relationship—requires balance between individuals
6	Jealousy: from/toward others
7	Possessiveness: from/toward others
8	Solvable/unsolvable
9	Thought pollution: from/toward others

Resolution for Relationship Issue

- Check the *Emotional Gauge for HHH Dowsing* p. 57.
- Consult other books, leaflets, etc. for material pertaining to relationship issues.

Sexual Issues and Resolutions

For more clues, check *Table of Contents* p. 86 for *Influences on Body-Mind-Spirit Issues.*

Person in the Relationship

1	Husband Wife Child Brother Sister Father Mother Son Daughter
2	Father-in-law Mother-in-law Son-in-law Daughter-in-law Aunt Uncle
3	Niece Nephew Cousin Grandfather Grandmother Granddaughter Grandson
4	Stepmother, father, daughter, son, brother, sister, etc.
5	Friend Acquaintance Stranger

Kind of Relationship or Problems with the Relationship

1	Too much Not enough Too painful No feelings
2	Frigid Impotent
3	Different styles, positions, pillow, devices, partners
4	Be conservative Be open minded
5	Oral Masturbation
6	Homosexuality: gay, lesbian Sex roles Sexual inequality
7	Abuse: rape, incest, molestation, verbal harassment
8	STD's (sexually transmitted diseases)--AIDS, gonorrhea, chlamydia, syphilis, herpes, infections (yeast, etc.)
9	Religious figure: priest, nun, pastor, deacon, etc.
10	Work-related Sexual discrimination Sexual harassment Coworker Boss
11	Health care setting: home care, nursing home, doctor, nurse, hospital
12	Locations: jail, school, other Law enforcement officer Social worker
13	Dressed too feminine/masculine Too much male energy / female energy
14	Imbalance in sexual energy Feel too feminine/too masculine Sexual energy and hormones
15	Different nature Different: culture, heritage, country, style, race, religious or belief, prejudice
16	Advanced sexual development/delayed sexual development Sex age: too old, too young
17	Possessiveness from/towards others Jealousy Fear Obsessive compulsive disorder
18	Stalking Can't relate to Check past lives.

Difference between Love and Lust

- Lust is wanting and consuming others (the body owns them).
- A lustful relationship emphasizes animalism, sensuality, concupiscence, sexuality.
- A loving relationships emphasize peace, harmony, understanding, caring, God, unconditional love.

Resolution for Sexual Issue

- Check the *Emotional Gauge for HHH Dowsing* p. 57.
- Consult other books, leaflets, etc. for material pertaining to sexual issues.

Social Issues, Table of Contents

Social Issues

For more clues, also check other books or resources; check other sections of *Table of Contents* p. 86 for *Influences on Body-Mind-Spirit Issues*; and check *Emotional Gauge for HHH Dowsing* p. 57.

Events that Can Cause the Issue

Abuse   Accident   Dis-ease   Misuse   Neglect   Operation   Shock   Trauma

Self Issues and Resolutions

1	Feelings Thoughts Emotions Psychological Pathological
2	Abuse: emotional, physical, mental, sexual, spiritual, financial
3	Suicidal Codependent Character traits: positive, negative
4	Social Antisocial Social task Counseling Sociopath Psychopath
5	Egotistical Discriminating Prejudiced Selfless
6	Lack of ego Lack self-confidence Feel accepted Feel unaccepted, humiliated, rejected, forlorn
7	Misunderstood Not prepared Misrepresented Mismanaged Manageable Movable
8	Self-word: education (self-education) esteem expression fulfillment limiting realization respect righteous sacrificing sufficient awareness assurance appraisal centered confidence control deceit discovery transformation
9	Serenity Setback Restructuring Laziness Temper
10	Temptation Sacrifice Communication Thought pollution from: self, others
11	Homeless Poverty stricken
12	Wealth: wealthy, too much, abuse of wealth
13	Abusers/users of people, of places, of others
14	Aggressive: a positive role, a negative role Passive: a positive role, a negative role
15	Phobias Compulsions Respected/not respected Fun to be with/not fun to be with
16	Passionate Laughing Love Romance Partnership Relationship

Resolutions for Self
- Place/niche in society: needs to find, needs to restructure, is inadequate, is adequate
- Should follow norms and rules
- Should not follow norms and rules (follow own drummer)
- Work to change society: from the outside, from the inside

Home Issues

1	Environment at birth Engagement Pregnancies Marriage
2	Divorce Changing family New partners Death Gender Retirement
3	Sex Roles Age (young, old) Discrimination
4	Household chores Loss of home, job, income
5	Important decisions: minor decisions/major decisions, business, professional, occupational

(continued)

Social Issues, continued

Schools/Education Institutions and People

1	Parochial Public
2	Preschool Head Start Kindergarten Primary Elementary Middle school Junior high
3	High school Trade school Vocational/technical College University Graduate school
4	Military academy Dance Music Art Sport Location of school Classes Semesters Quarters
6	School people: Superintendent Principal Professor Teacher Aide Guidance counselor Students Custodian Janitor Secretary Kitchen workers Student teacher Librarian

Business Occupations and Resolutions

Occupations, professions, and possible positions and resolutions are listed below.

1	Business management Marketing Financing Corporation Corporate power CEO Secretary
2	Executives Accounting Assessor/controller/treasurer Technological advice
3	Engineering: mechanical, electrical, civil, industrial
4	Applied computer technology Computer programming: personal computer, business computer
5	Specialist: computer-assisted bookkeeping, PC repair Desktop publishing
6	Medical office assistant Dental assistant Medical transcriptionist Counselor Doctor (many types)
7	Psychiatrist Psychologist Gun repair Locksmith Punch press
8	Auto mechanic Motor cycle repair Drafting Animal care specialist Travel agent
9	Florist Assembler Freight Sales Tax preparation Crafts Funeral director
10	Police science Private security officer Police Detective Fire fighter Legal assistant
11	Art: painting, drawing, sculpting Photographer Photography Model Actress/actor
12	Farmer Conservation Wildlife management Forestry management Surveying/mapping
13	Design Interior decorating Catering: gourmet cooking, cafeteria Fitness Nutrition
14	Dressmaking/design Real estate appraiser Home inspector TV/VCR repair Appliance repair
15	Teacher's Aide Child day care provider/owner Journalism Short story writing
16	Hotel/restaurant management Hospitality management Dishwasher Waitress
17	Pattern maker Model maker Papermaker Interviewer Recreation
18	Air-conditioning/heating and refrigeration Construction worker Carpenter Slater Roofer Lather
19	Electrician Excavation Brick mason Stone mason Cement finisher Drywall installer
20	International/overseas Small business/large business Small business management

Resolutions for Business

- Both members of family should work: mother/father
- Not capable of organizing a business
- Should own and run own business
- Should have partner/should change partner
- Change business: close, relocate, add on to, streamline
- One parent needs to stay home for children
- Highly capable to organize and run a business
- Use business to help community
- Be careful with choosing customers/partners
- Advertising: need to do it, change tactics
- Suitable or right livelihood (Are you creating negativity, dishonesty, exploitation through your livelihood? Employment should not create paranoia and separateness in the world.)

(continued)

Social Issues, continued

Government/Political Institutions and Ideas and Resolutions

1	Federal State County Municipal
2	Political departments: presidential, senator, congressman, mayor, alderman, judicial, diplomat, ambassador, foreign affairs
3	Orientation: radical, liberal, conservative, reactionary, activist, pacifist
4	Military: Navy, Army, Marines, Air Force, Coast Guard, National Guard
5	Military draft Draft dodger
6	Law enforcement: CIA, FBI, Secret Service, sheriff, deputy, police officer, truant officer
7	Social service Health department
8	Legal system: courts (Supreme-federal, state, district, circuit, appeals), judge, jury, prosecutor, defense attorney, bailiff
9	Social services: case worker, rules, regulations
10	Post Office
11	Medicare Medicaid Medical Assistance
12	Chamber of Commerce City hall
13	Patents Inventions
14	Population change: emigration, immigration (legal, illegal)
15	Political awareness and movements: American Civil Liberties Union, NAACP

Resolutions for Political Issues

- Enter politics.
- Avoid politics.
- Become politically aware.
- Attempt to change politics/government.
- Become a part of a political or governmental movement.
- Become conscious of world, national, state and local government and politics.

Agencies (Financial, Real Estate, Insurance, Sales)

1	Sales/service: realtors, insurance (car, home, business, health, life), travel, job service, employment.
2	Advertising, modeling.
3	See also *Business Occupations and Resolutions* p. 97.

(continued)

Social Issues, continued

Social/Health Clubs and Organizations and Resolutions

1	Military clubs, organizations
2	Civic clubs, organizations: Moose, Elk, NOW, Lions, Rotary, Shriners, Boys and Girls, Eastern Star, YMCA, YWCA, Boy and Girl Scouts,
3	Fitness: athletic organization, health, nutrition, weight loss, exercise
4	Nonprofit organizations: Red Cross, Salvation Army, Heart and Lung Assoc., March of Dimes, AIDS victim support, Assoc. for Retarded Persons

Resolutions

- Join a club or organization.
- A club/organization is helpful/harmful.
- Financially support a club/organization.
- Become an active member of a club/organization.

Media and Resolutions

1	News Newspaper News media Public relations Films Magazines Books
2	Advertising Yellow Pages Radio TV VCR Cassette tapes Telephone
3	Computer (Internet and World Wide Web) Weather broadcasting Mail
4	Subliminal media: messages, programming, suggestions, control, thoughts

Resolutions about Media

- Make use of media.
- Avoid media.
- Find a job in media.
- Incorporate media into one's life and/or business.
- Use media as a way of spreading your message.
- Be aware of media abuse (on part of politicians, wealthy, public, etc.

Sports, Games, and other Leisure Activities

1	Baseball Football Basketball Hockey Soccer Golf Martial arts Rugby Aerobics
2	Swimming Ice skating Rollerskating Fencing Sailing Boating Dancing
3	Chess Cards Board games Reading Singing Writing Art and art related Gambling
4	Horse racing Skiing Hiking Backpacking Biking Walking Exploring Bird watching etc.

Resolutions about Sports, Games, Leisure Activities

- Find leisure time activities.
- Find new source of recreational activities.
- Find physical activities.
- Have fewer sport or leisure activities.
- Stop sports activities.

(continued)

Social Issues, continued

Medical/Healthcare/Human–Animal Research–Development

1	Institution: hospital, retirement home, foster home, group home, nursing home, skilled care home, research facility, handicapped facility, institution for mentally ill
2	Animal shelter
3	Financed: independent, private, government sponsored, community sponsored
4	Practitioners: doctor, family, surgeon, chiropractor, psychiatrist, optometrist, nurse, hygienist, dietitian, veterinarian
5	Medical instrument: doctor, dentist, optometrist, etc.

Resolutions

- Find appropriate medical care.
- Find a different doctor or medical practitioner.
- Consult for second opinion.
- Find an alternative facility.
- Look for a pet at animal shelter.
- There are/check for problems with doctor or other medical practitioner.
- Consider placement in home or facility.
- Remove the being from facility or home.
- A human/animal is receiving improper treatment/proper treatment.

(continued)

Social Issues, continued

Monetary Establishments

1	Bank system: officers, tellers, world banks, national banks, Federal Reserve, IRS, state banks, credit unions, savings and loan
2	Alternate sources: check-cashing facilities, loan shark, investment brokers, stockbrokers, accountant, secretary
3	Accounts: checking, savings, bonds, certificates of deposit, money market funds, stocks, commodities, IRA, tax sheltered annuities

Resolutions Involving Monetary Establishments

- Find an appropriate financial institution to hold your money.
- Change banks.
- Withdraw and invest money.
- Consult an accountant.
- Money may be improperly invested.
- Use money for charitable organizations or reasons.

Religions/Religious Institutions

1	Place of worship: church, synagogue, temple, mosque, nature, altar, within self, outside of self
2	Religious service: traditional, free form
3	Clergy: deacon, priest, nun, monk, priest, pastor, rabbi, pope, bishop, cardinal, preacher
4	Ladies/men aid clubs, choir, Bible study group
5	Religious schools/academies See different religious beliefs and practices (some are listed on p. 75).

Resolutions

- Seek different church or place of worship.
- There are/check for problems with leaders or members or your church religious group.
- Find an appropriate religious setting.
- Change/join religious group or club to help in your seeking and fulfillment.
- Consider alternative approaches to religion and the spiritual life.

Technology and Technological Developments

1	Advances in computers Medical technology	
2	Space technology Military weapons Communications	

Resolutions

- Acknowledge/remove fear of technology.
- Become involved with technology.
- Avoid technology.
- Make use of new technology.
- Become part of technological developments.

Social Issues, continued

Places, Space, Travel, and Transportation Issues and Resolutions

1	Mode of travel: Car Truck Motorcycle Scooter Moped Bicycle Airline Horse Covered wagon On foot Company Transport Train Camper Tent Caravan Mobile home Recreational vehicle Sailboat Yacht Motorboat Tugboat Barge Bus Tourism Cruise
2	Where: Hall Boat Apartment Guest house Hotel Business Property Garden Land Cottage House Home (yours/others) Food Establishment Highway Road Museum Low/high mountains Hills Plateau Marsh Sea Dunes Beach Forest Lake Desert Bath Health spa Island Market Building Farm Community Village Town Urban area City Country Nation State County Township

Resolutions

- Change mode of transportation.
- Keep mode of transportation.
- Travel.
- Remain home.
- Take a vacation.
- Move to new residence.

Culture, Race, or Ethnic Issues and Resolutions

1	Cultural: similarity, difference, clash, unity
2	Race or skin color: Black White Brown Yellow Caucasian Negroid Hispanic Native American Asian
3	Interracial Intracultural Biracial
4	Interfaith Prejudice Discrimination Minority Immigrant

Resolutions

- Be open to other cultural experiences.
- There is/check for a form of prejudice/discrimination.
- Afraid of (*fill in your personal statement here*).
- Remember past immigration of relatives.
- Avoid certain cultural/ethnic/racial clashes.

(continued)

Social Issues, continued

Violence/Crime Issues and Resolutions

1	Fire—arson Vandalism Threats Forgery Destructiveness Assassination
2	Riots Burglary Assault Rape Murder Theft Libel Slander Insults War
3	Breaking and entering Weapons: guns, knives, explosives, poisons
4	Criminal behavior Mafia Underworld Black market
5	Prison Jail Concentration camps

Resolutions

- Be aware of potential problems from others.
- Avoid certain areas of country, city, town, neighborhood.
- Do not consider violent/criminal behavior.
- Use violence as a last resort.

Holidays/Special Calendar Events and Resolutions

1	New Years Eve/Day Valentine's Day Easter Passover Palm Sunday
2	Presidents' birthdays Memorial Day Veteran's Day
3	Armistice Day Pearl Harbor Day Independence Day (July 4)
4	Mother's Day Father's Day Grandparent's Day Secretary's Day
5	Halloween All Saint's Eve Thanksgiving Christmas Hanukah
6	Family birthday's Anniversary Graduation Confirmation
7	Marriage Engagement Family death days
8	By ethnic or religious group: African Jewish European Indian Asian Native American Australian Pagan Satanic Christian

Resolution

- A specific day causes turmoil, depression, happiness.
- Reevaluate the meaning or significance of a specific day or holiday.
- Celebrate/stop celebrating.
- Mourn/stop mourning.
- Remember and acknowledge/need to forget.

SUPPORTING MATERIAL

Table of Contents

Supplementary Pages to Tear Out
    Body Chart (two sheets)
    Imbalance/Issue Record Sheet (two sheets)
    Emotional Gauge for HHH Dowsing (one sheet)

Resolutions

The following statements, goals, etc., are potential tools for the process of healing. Dowsing or scanning through these might give you a clue as to things that need to be said or done to help in the process of healing. **The most important however, is to let go and resolve your issues by writing things out on paper, and to then send a blessing or love with it; for more information, see step 12 on p. 35.**

‖   Love is the greatest power in the universe.   ‖

Blessings

The Power of Blessing

When you have problems with bad things, bless the good things in your life.

Perfect love casts out all fears.

Believe that you are healed.

I am a channel of Divine Love.

What to Bless

Bless: Love, God, Light and Love, Perfect Living, Your Soul, The Higher Self, Perfect Love, Beauty, Energy, Balance, Breath, Life, Death, Awakening, Harmony, I am One, Oneness, Peace, Stability, Hope, Life-force, the Lord

Statements of Blessing

Bless with Universal Love.

Bless all levels of Love, Bless Love on all levels.

I am present, I come with love, I depart with love.

I am at peace with (*insert your personal statement here*).

May the Creator of the Universal Law bless us.

Bless this person today so he/she is clear of (*insert your personal statement here*).

Please bless my body for the next 24 hours so it is clean of negative thought forms, psychic, physical, emotional, and mental attacks.

Resolutions, continued

Cleansing

Blow or brush over skin/object/body to remove impurities, blockages, etc.

Burn incense.

Use smudging.

Place object or self in sunlight.

You may also use salt, water, herbs, spices, flowers, oils, etc. in the process of cleansing. It often is good to use visualization or verbalization during the process to help with the cleansing. Many people perform it as a ritual or ceremony to add strength to the process.

Thoughts, Affirmations, Statements

> We create our own story by our thoughts and actions. What we think and feel in our mind and heart, we will produce in our experience and our life. What we give, we get. As within, so without.

Everything is in divine order for my Highest Good!

Everything is taken care of in its own time.

I am in harmony with the good in all portions of my life.

I breathe in power and exhale love.

I now seal and heal my aura from all outside influences. The Spirit of God is in me now.

I am happy forever. Nothing hinders me.

> I walk with Beauty (God) before me.
> I walk with Beauty (God) behind me.
> I walk with Beauty (God) above me.
> I walk with Beauty (God) below me.
> I walk with Beauty (God) around me.
> Native American prayer

My (God's) words are beautiful.

I am a Channel of Divine Love.

I am receptive to the love of God.

I am real, myself.

God is in me.

(continued)

Resolutions and **Thoughts, Affirmations, Statements,** continued

I am ready to follow God and his/her/its will.

I am reliable for God.

My choices brought me to where I am, and I am responsible for my life.

‖   "Ask" and it will be given.   ‖
                    "Seek" and you will find.
                           "Knock" and it shall be opened to you.

Make a short list of those things in your life that you need to give up. Then decide which is most important to let go, and then go to work on letting it go.

No matter where you come from, you're always going somewhere.

Do not judge or ridicule anyone until you have walked in their shoes.

Celebrate your life. See yourself as getting better and wiser rather than just getting older.

‖   Say yes to yourself.   ‖
                   Be honest to yourself.
                       Surprise yourself.

Resolutions and **Thoughts, Affirmations, Statements,** continued

The following is based on material put together by Rill Delaney:

1. Think good, and good follows. Think evil, and evil follows. You are what you think all day long.

2. Your subconscious mind does not argue with you. It accepts what your conscious mind decrees. If you think "I can't afford it," it may be true, but do not say it. Select a better thought decree " I can buy it," or "I accept it in my mind."

3. You have the power to choose. Choose health and happiness. You can choose to be friendly, or you can choose to be unfriendly. You can choose to be cooperative, joyous, friendly, lovable, and the whole world responds. This is the best way to develop a wonderful personality.

4. Your conscious mind is the "watchman at the gate." Its chief function is to protect our subconscious mind from false impressions. Choose to believe that something good can happen and it is happening now. Your greatest power is your capacity to choose. Choose happiness and abundance.

5. The suggestions and statements of others have no power to hurt you. The only power is the movement of your own thought. You can choose to reject the thoughts or statements of others and affirm the good. You have the power to choose how you react.

6. Watch what you say. You have to account for every idle word. Never say "I will fail, I will lose my job, I can't pay the rent." Your subconscious cannot take a joke. It brings all these things to pass.

7. Your mind is not evil. No force of nature is evil. It depends on how you use the powers of nature. Use your mind to bless, heal, and inspire all people everywhere.

8. Never say that you can't overcome fear. Substitute the following sentence: "I can do all things through the power of my own subconscious mind."

9. Begin to think from the standpoint of the eternal truth and principles of life, and not from the standpoint of fear, ignorance, and superstition. Do not let others do your thinking for you. Choose your own thoughts and make your own decisions.

Resolutions, continued

Forgiveness

Forgiveness is an important process to be incorporated in your growth. If things and/or people are not forgiven, they lie hidden and store anger and resentment. This is not beneficial to your growth and development. It is important to consciously work on forgiveness and acceptance of others. In this process you will free yourself from ties that would otherwise hold you back. Here are example affirmations:

> From this moment on, I forgive this person for what he/she has done to me. I wish him/her well. I may want no further association with him/her, but I hereafter refuse to permit thoughts of this person to upset me emotionally, or to affect my health, happiness and harmony.

> I forgive this person as I hope to be forgiven for my part in this misunderstanding. I know that as I remove all feelings of hate and resentment, the way will be open for new understanding because like attracts like, and my changed attitude must attract a changed attitude in return.

Life Pattern Changes

To yield to God.   To trust others.   To trust God.

To recognize when it is appropriate to trust.

To be wise.   To be peaceful.

To be in harmony with God, the universe, and nature.

To be pleasing to God.   To be honest.   To see the truth.

To love and obey God.   To have wisdom and vision.

To hear God and the Universe.   To know the truth.

To be at peace and harmony.   To be content and blessed.

To be peaceful.   To have faith.   To rely on God.

To love others as myself.   To have joy.   To give thanks.

To allow God to use me.   To be patient.   To have self control.

To be gentle.   To overcome.   To forgive myself, to forgive others.

To forget the past.   To be kind.   To be tactful.

To have my spirits high.   To have vision.

(continued)

Resolutions and **Life Pattern Changes**, continued

To attract positive influences.   To choose relationships that help me mature.

To choose wisely.   To welcome beneficial change.

My inner wisdom is guiding me now.   To be humble.

To be meek.   To be tolerant.   To be modest.   To be free.

To be thankful for spiritual guidance.   To ask for spiritual guidance.

Use waiting time for God. While waiting in line, for service etc. say prayers, give thanks, ask for guidance.

Count your blessings. Give thanks for little miracles. Note the good things that are part of your hectic life.

Take responsibility for your own spiritual life or path.

Explore what spirituality means to you. Find a spiritual community. Find a spiritual director (one who is of the same sex who you can talk to more openly).

Take time to be quiet, meditate, do yoga, pray. Make your best effort to do it the same time everyday.

Make a prayer/meditation corner.

Read spiritual material: Bible verses, devotional.

Keep a prayer diary. Write your own Psalms.

Work for justice and human rights.

Help the poor and homeless.

Help the people on your path. Remember those on the margin.

Pray for others.

Always plan to be kind.

Make amends.

Guard your tongue.

Practice appreciation.

Work for a more peaceful world.

Celebrate creation. Restore God's creation.

Pay attention to your own dreams.

(continued)

Resolutions and **Life Pattern Changes**, continued

Speak of spiritual things with your family.

Clean your house physically and spiritually. As you clean, look for things you no longer need that you can share with those that are in need.

Be a child again (childlike, not childish). See the uniqueness and beauty in everything.

Learn to again appreciate the simple things in life.

Don't fear the future. Live life as it comes and realize things that need to be changed and those that cannot be changed. Live one day at a time. The only time you really have is **now**.

Be friendly, joyful. Wear a smile, even when it is hard to do so. Accept your burdens with a joy for a lesson to be learned from which you will grow and mature. Have a sense of humor.

Be thankful for what you have. Avoid greed and materialism. Don't collect more than you need, for ultimately the possessions will become burdens.

Keep positive thoughts in your head. Negative thoughts become burdens and painful weapons that will eventually turn on you.

Accept criticism without letting it tear into you. Often it may just as easily be dismissed, for the criticism that is given to you is actually meant for the persons themselves (their own insecurity, frustration, fear, resentment, etc.).

Organize yourself. Set priorities and goals that are reasonable and uplifting to your life and growth.

Be honest with yourself. Admit and realize when you are wrong, but don't be guilty or ashamed of your mistakes.

Be yourself. Don't try to impress others by being someone or something that you are not.

Take care of yourself physically, spiritually, emotionally, mentally. Be at peace with yourself.

Proper Self-talk:
Do you hear what you said?
Why did you do this to me? They would not have done it if you would not have allowed it.

Resolutions, continued

Colors

Colors may be used to stimulate, calm down, balance, etc. They may be worn as clothing, painted on walls, held, looked at, visualized, colored, or drawn with. To find further information, consult texts or specific books that deal with color therapy.

1	Make use of	Do not use	Avoid	Cover with						
2	Full Color	Shades	Tints	Transparent	Opaque					
3	Red	Orange	Yellow	Green	Blue	Indigo	Violet	Black	Brown	White	Gray

Gemstones/Minerals

Gems, rocks, and minerals have been used by people for hundreds of thousands of years and in many ways. Some cultures believe they have certain properties that can assist a person in their daily life, not merely as colorful adornment or as decorations. The past decade has brought forth a great number of books which discuss the various properties of the rocks and gems. If you are attracted to this method of healing (e.g. gemstone therapy), consult the variety of texts that are available for more information. You will be surprised at the great variety of stones available. They have a rainbow of colors, textures, luster, etc., that can be helpful to you or others.

1	Make use of gemstones.	Avoid gemstones.		
2	Purchase gemstones.	Find your own gemstones.	Receive gemstones as gifts.	Give gemstone gifts.

Music

Music has been around as long as human kind has existed, if not longer. Here again we suggest you consult various texts and materials to find a type of music or a method of music therapy that might be most beneficial to you. The list of chakras in *Locations of the Seven Main Centers* p. 74, give notes of the musical scale corresponding to chakras and consequently to various organs of the body. Certain instruments also correspond to certain parts of the body and will stimulate its various parts.

Be aware of feelings that occur in your body and mind while listening to music. Feel vibrations and moods that occur. Be careful of the lyrics that might accompany the music as well. Remember that words have a direct effect on the way we act and feel.

1	Listen to/avoid: classical rock country blues rap soul instrumental vocal chanting drumming pop opera New Age.
2	Play a musical instrument. Use your voice to sing or hum. Write your own music lyrics.
3	Feel, integrate, and express healing vibration in movement.
4	Use music: daily weekly monthly.
5	Music is the soundtrack of your life.

Resolutions, continued

Symbols

People have used symbols and signs throughout their existence. Many symbols have an extensive history behind them. For example, the Christian cross was in use long before the religion of Christianity was in existence.

You can find it beneficial to incorporate symbols in your life to help in cleansing, focusing, healing, clearing, remembering, etc. There are several texts available to consult that can help in your search to find appropriate symbols to incorporate in your life. Others can search for symbols that should be avoided.

1	Symbol has a negative, draining effect.
2	Symbol has an uplifting, enlightening effect.
3	Symbol should be avoided / incorporated in one's life.
4	Create your own symbol.
5	Explore the meaning of the symbols that attract you or make you feel uncomfortable.

Nature

Make use of animals, plants, insects, climate (clouds, thunderstorms, weather phenomena), the earth and earth forces. Many people can tune into the various aspects of nature and receive lessons, energy, insight, power, etc. Native American materials are becoming more available. Lost lessons are resurfacing, giving us insights into what can be learned from our brothers, sisters, aunts, uncles and all relations in the natural world. Be open to these things as they are a part of us and we are a part of them.

1	Listen to nature. Sit in natural settings.
2	Study certain plants, animals, natural phenomena.
3	Restore or create natural settings around you.
4	Provide money for nature preservation.
5	Become an activist for natural causes.
6	Take walks or hikes in nature.
7	Do not disrupt nature.
8	Repair a natural setting by reintroducing native species to the area.
9	Inspire children, neighbors, schools, others to become aware of the nature around them.

Resolutions, continued
Life Lessons

> The past is history.
> The future a mystery.
> The present is a gift from God.
> Live today.
>
> When our lessons are finished we "graduate."

> All the hardships that you face in life, all the tests and tribulations, all the nightmares and all the losses, most people still view as curses, as punishments by God, as something negative. If you would only know that nothing that comes to you is negative. I mean nothing.
>
> All the trials and tribulations, and the biggest losses that you ever experienced, things that make you say "If I had only known about this, I would never have been able to make it through", are gifts to you. It's like somebody has to—what do you call that when you make the hot iron into a tool?—you have to temper the iron.
>
> It is an opportunity that you are given to grow. That is the whole purpose of existence on this planet earth. You will not grow if you sit in a beautiful flower garden and somebody brings you gorgeous food on a silver platter. But you will grow if you are sick, if you are in pain, if you experience losses, and if you do not put your head in the sand, but take the pain and learn to accept it, not as a curse or punishment, but as a gift to you with a very, very specific purpose.
>
> Elisabeth Kübler-Ross
> **Death Does Not Exist**

Free Forever Formula

> Positive "F" Words:
> The Free Forever Formula

> To have **f**reedom means to "move **f**orward" by **f**orgiving, **f**orgetting, and being **f**ulfilled. Also, you need to **f**eel **f**ortunate and to be **f**illed with **f**aith. Build a strong **f**oundation **f**or the **f**uture without **f**ear or **f**riction. Allow yourself to **f**eel the **f**reedom of your soul in **f**light.
> Doris Hagemann and Anneliese Hagemann

For more information, consult books and references. Also, check *Conventional and Holistic Healing Methods for Body-Mind-Spirit* on p. 19.

References

The following list is only a glimpse at possible reference materials that can be helpful in your search for information and methods to deal with issues. There is no way that we could truly put together a comprehensive list. Consult libraries, health food stores, new age stores, friends, and acquaintances for more information. You can find many different approaches and ideas that don't always agree with one another. Thus it is up to you to find the path or approach that most suits your way of interpreting and dealing with things. Good luck in your search.

Resources from Anneliese Gabriel Hagemann

Anneliese has published the following books:
A Quick Gauge to Body-Mind-Spirit Wellness Immune System Balancer
Dowsing/Divining the Golden Key to Tapping Energies
Guidelines for Living in Your Divine Truth
Search for My Life's Path/Soul Mission
Spiritual Enlightenment
To Our Health

Anneliese teaches the following classes:
- Facilitator training class, which includes all the books listed above.
- Dowsing class, which includes the Workbook titled To Our Health: Using the Inner Art of Dowsing in the Search for Health-Happiness-Harmony in Body-Mind-Spirit.

Other Books, by Author's Last Name or by Publisher

Carol Bridges: The Medicine Woman Inner Guidebook
Hugh Burroughs: Alternative Healing: 160 different healing methods
Hulda Regehr Clark Ph.D., M.D.: The Cure for HIV and AIDS
Harvey and Marilyn Diamond: Fit for Life
Lee DuBelle: Proper Food Combination Works
Ona C. Evers: Everybody's Dowsers Book
Ada P. Kahn and Linda Hughes Holt, M.D.: Mid Life Health
Biokinesiology Institute: Muscle Testing
W. J. "Rill" Finch: The Pendulum and Possession
Holy Bible (see especially: Corinthians Chapter 11 - 14)
Beatrice Trum Hunters: Additive Book
Leslie J. Kaslof: The Traditional Flower Remedies of Dr. Bach
(continued)

References, continued

.Jethro Kloss: <u>Back to Eden</u>

Rev. Hanna Kroeger: <u>Ageless Remedies from Mother's Kitchen</u>

Rev. Hanna Kroeger: <u>God Helps Those That Help Themselves</u>

Rev. Hanna Kroeger: <u>Parasites, The Enemy Within</u>

Rev. Hanna Kroeger: <u>The Pendulum The Bible and Your Survival</u>

Rev. Hanna Kroeger: <u>Seven Spiritual Causes of Ill Health</u>

Rev. Hanna Kroeger: <u>New Dimensions in Healing Yourself</u> (also in video)

Rev. Hanna Kroeger: <u>Cancer- Traditional and New Concepts</u>

Louise L. Hay: <u>You Can Heal Your Body</u>

Louise L. Hay: <u>You Can Heal Your Life</u>

Ted J. Kaptchuk: <u>The Web That Has No Weaver</u> (Chinese Medicine)

Reba Ann Karp: <u>Edgar Cayce- Encyclopedia of Healing</u>

Elisabeth Kübler-Ross: <u>Death and Dying</u>

John Lust: <u>The Herb Book</u>

Bote Mikkers: <u>The Pendulum Workbook</u>

Marlo Morgan: <u>Mutant Message Down Under</u>

Melody: <u>Love is in the Earth (A guide to gemstones and their uses)</u>

Greg Nielson and Joseph Polansky: <u>Pendulum Power</u>

Greg Nielson: <u>Beyond Pendulum Power</u>

Ocean Tree Books Santa Fe, NM: <u>Peace Pilgrim</u>

Dr. Dean Ornish: <u>Dr. Dean Ornish's Program for Reversing Heart Disease</u>

Jeannine Parvati: Hygieia: <u>A Woman's Herbal</u>

Genevieve Lewis Paulson: <u>Kundalini and the Chakras</u>

Sara Shannon: <u>Diet for the Atomic Age</u>

Mary Summer Rain: <u>Earthway</u>

John F.Thie, D.C.: <u>Touch for Health: A new approach to restore our natural energies</u>

Barbara G. Walker: <u>The Women's Dictionary of Symbols and Sacred Objects</u>

Gordon Stokes and Daniel Whiteside: <u>The Behavior Barometer's World</u>

Chelsea Yarbro: <u>Messages from Michael</u>

Conclusion

As we finalized this book, we realized more than ever that it will always be incomplete. There is no way it can ever be complete. The world and universe are constantly changing and growing. Things will always need to be added. This we leave to you, the reader and user of this material.

We hope you have found this book a help in your search to achieve some balance in your life. If you feel that we have missed something important, or if you wish to further add to or discuss a portion of this material, feel free to contact us. We welcome and are open to any new insights and ideas.

Peace and Love
Anneliese Hagemann and Doris Hagemann

A few comments from the HHH Dowsing Workshop Questionnaire about the workshop and the presenter, Anneliese Gabriel Hagemann:

<u>What do you feel were the most beneficial things you learned from the workshop?</u>

"Healing--It's for everyone, and it is simple. It was a WOW class. Hope our paths cross again."
Betty Westphal

"That your body does not lie--Trust that source of information. I learned so many important aspects about myself, which allows me to grow, because I felt I was stuck. You are truly a miracle. Thank you so much for coming in my life. You are a true inspiration Dr. Oma. Bless Love. Bless Love."
Kirsten Severed

"The importance of separating ego from self, to be able to use the Art of Dowsing."
Mary Hannigan

"How to use dowsing to help myself and others. The workshop was wonderful."
Lynne Zawojski

"I have the tools to be in control of my life--future--and spirit. All I need to do is ask myself."
Jeff Peterson

"How my body is affected by issues that my conscious mind does not even acknowledge."
Patti Miller

INDEX

- A -

angels described, 83
aura
  colors of, 71
  description of, 69
  layers described, 70
  listed on Body Chart, 17

- B -

Bless Love
  example prayers using, 7, 81
  example resolutions using, 36, 85, 105
  purpose, 36
  to balance an issue 100%, 37
Body Chart
  chakras described, 73, 74
  example, 17
  instructions to use it, 22
  layers of aura described, 70
  soul levels described, 84
Body issues - list of influences, 24, 39
Body-Mind-Spirit
  interconnectedness, 1, 24
  list of influences, 24
Body-Mind-Spirit influences - list of, 86

- C -

chakras
  colors associated with, 57, 74
  description of, 73
  emotions/attitudes associated with, 57, 74
  list of, 57, 74
  listed on Body Chart, 17
  musical notes associated with, 74
  problems with, 74
chi
  description of, 73
  problems with, 74
conventional healing methods
  dowsing for, 14
  list of, 19
crawl-in soul, 80

- D -

dowsing
  ancient art of, 2
  asking guidance for, 7, 14
  asking permission for, 7, 14, 84
  drinking water before, 8
  guidelines, 7
  Highest Good as the intention, 3, 10, 13
  indicator of human nervous system, 2
  learning to use pendulum, 9
  phrasing a question for, 8
  Thank you at end of session, 10, 11, 37
  to identify a problem, 2
  tools for, 3, 10, 11
  using the word "Suppress", 37
  using this Workbook, 5

- E -

Emotional Gauge for HHH Dowsing
  description of, 57
  to help identify issues, 24, 34, 96
  to help resolve issues, 62, 90, 93, 94
emotions or energy
  negative, 57, 58, 59, 60, 61
  positive, 57, 63

- F -

forgiveness
  a Law of Universal Consciousness, 84
  and karma, 77
  prayers, affirmations, 81, 109
Free Forever Formula, 114

- G -

guidelines for dowsing
  instructions, 7
  summary, 5

- H -

healing
  and achieving balance, 1
  method, dowsing for, 14
  methods, conventional, 19
  methods, holistic, 19
health, definition of, 1

Highest Good
  as intention of dowsing, 3, 7, 13
  dowsing tool for, 10, 11
  goals in support of, 37
  to express a resolution, 35, 106
holistic healing methods
  dowsing for, 14
  list of, 19

- I -

Imbalance/Issue Record Sheet
  example, 18
  irecording step 13, 37
  recording item 1.A,1.B, 14
  recording item 1.C, 14
  recording step 10, 31
  recording step 11, 34
  recording step 12, 35
  recording step 2, 22
  recording step 3, 23
  recording step 4, 23
  recording step 5, 24
  recording step 7, 28
  recording step 8, 26, 29
  recording step 9, 30
immune system
  balancing - book by Anneliese Hagemann, 115
  components of, 26
  manifests an issue with the body, 54
  manifests an issue with the mind, 66
issues,
  See also resolutions
  acid-alkaline balance as cause of, 52
  afflictions resulting from attachments, 80
  allergies - symptoms, 42
  as life lessons, 84, 114
  atmospheric causes of, 44
  aura influences on, 72
  behavioral concerns, 88
  belief systems as influence on, 76
  brain's four layers – list of, 55
  business occupations related to, 97
  carbohydrates as causes of, *See* books about nutrition
  chemical causes of, 45
  chi problems, 74
  childhood diseases as causes of, 55
  cultural influences on, 102
  drugs and treatments as causes of, 46
  educational, 87, 97
  electrical influences on, 49
  electromagnetic influences on, 49

Body Chart

① Name _____

Birth date _____

Goals to work on if no issues
show up _____

How many issues on the same spot? _____

② Conventional or holistic
healing method (pp. 19-21)

_____

_____

(If not enough room, record on
a separate piece of paper.)

③ Steps 2, 3, 4 (pp. 22, 23) on the *Imbalance / Issue Record*

Sheet: Most important issue; aura layer; level of
consciousness; amount of stress (Major, Major/Minor, etc.)

Major: _____

Major/Minor: _____

Minor: _____

Minor/Minor: _____

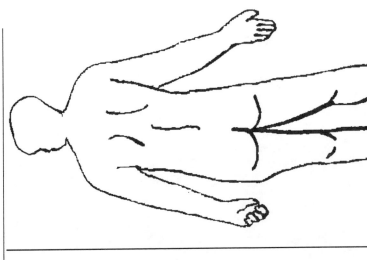

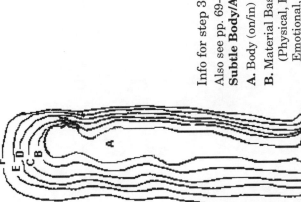

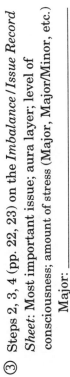

Info for step 2

Also see
pp. 73-74

**The Seven Major
Chakras**

1. Root
2. Sex
3. Solar Plexus
4. Heart
5. Throat
6. Third Eye
7. Crown
(8. New Brain)

Info for step 3

Also see pp. 69-70

Subtle Body/Aura Layers

A. Body (on/in)

B. Material Base Aspect
(Physical, Etheric,
Emotional, Mental)

C. Fulcrum Aspect

D. Individual Soul Aspect
(Etheric template,
Celestial; Ketheric, Auric)

E. God Force Aspect
(1st, 2nd Cosmic Bodies,
God/Tao Body)

F. Soul-Higher Soul Self

- See step 2 page 22 for instructions to fill in this *Body Chart.*
- Transfer information from this page to column for step 2 on the *Imbalance / Issue Record Sheet* on page 18.

Body Chart

① Name _____

Birth date _____

Goals to work on if no issues
show up _____

How many issues on the same spot? _____

② Conventional or holistic
healing method (pp. 19-21)

(If not enough room, record on
a separate piece of paper.)

③ Steps 2, 3, 4 (pp. 22, 23) on the *Imbalance/Issue Record Sheet*: Most important issue; aura layer; level of consciousness; amount of stress (Major, Major/Minor, etc.)

Major: _____

Major/Minor: _____

Minor: _____

Minor/Minor: _____

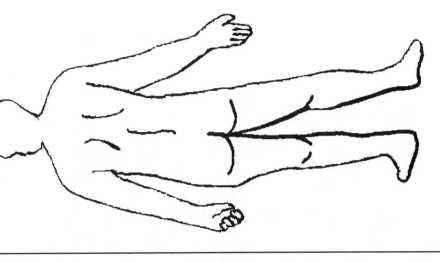

Info for step 3
Also see pp. 69-70
Subtle Body/Aura Layers

A. Body (on/in)
B. Material Base Aspect
   (Physical, Etheric,
   Emotional, Mental)
C. Fulcrum Aspect
D. Individual Soul Aspect
   (Etheric template,
   Celestial; Ketheric, Auric)
E. God Force Aspect
   (1st, 2nd Cosmic Bodies,
   God/Tao Body)
F. Soul-Higher Soul Self

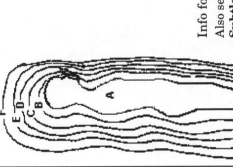

Info for step 2
Also see
pp. 73-74
**The Seven Major
Chakras**

1. Root
2. Sex
3. Solar Plexus
4. Heart
5. Throat
6. Third Eye
7. Crown
(8. New Brain)

• See step 2 page 22 for instructions to fill in this *Body Chart*.
• Transfer information from this page to column for step 2 on the *Imbalance/Issue Record Sheet* on page 18.

Imbalance/Issue Record Sheet

Name _____ Birth date _____ Address _____ Phone _____ .

☐ Step #1.A (p. 14)   #1.B What Method(s) are beneficial? _____ (p. 14)   #1.C Overall % balance. Before session: _____ After session: _____

Step 2 p. 22	Step 3 p. 23 Level: c sb sp unc du soul	Step 4 p. 23 Stress M, M/m, m, m/m	Step 5 p. 24 Ident. b, m, s, b/m/s	Step 6 p. 26 Manife-station	Step 7 p. 27 Who is in-volved?	Step 8 p. 29 Time	Step 9 p. 30 Origin	Step 10 p. 31 Clues	Step 11 p. 34 Emotional Gauge for HHH Dowsing Negative pp. 57, 58	Positive pp. 57, 63	Step 12 pp. 36, 105-114 Resolution	Step 13 p. 37 Always balance 100%
E	sb	M (Major)	M (Mind)	Central Nervous System	Friend Not my issue	About 2 monhs ago	My yard		Frustrated	Need to provide an ear	This is not my issue. I let go of the frustrated Energy which is held on my Subconscious level of my Being manifesting in my Central Nervous System. This energy no longer serves me. I provide an ear to listen to my friend Maxine. Thank You. Bless Love, Bless Love, Bless Love.	100%

for Step 3: c=conscious, sb=subconscious, sp=super-conscious, unc=unconscious, du=DUPI, soul=soul, ch=chosen, nc=not chosen

for Step 4: How much stress is involved: M=Major issue, M/m=Major/Minor issue, m=Minor issue, m/m=Minor/Minor issue

for step 5: b=body, m=mind, s=spirit, b/m/s=body and mind and spirit, o/u=Other or Unknown at this time

Imbalance/Issue Record Sheet

Name _____ Birth date _____ Phone _____ .

☐ Step #1.A (p. 14) | #1.B What Method(s) are beneficial? (p. 14) | #1.C Overall % balance. Before session: _____ (p. 14) After session: _____

Step 2 p. 22	Step 3 p. 23 Level: c sb sp unc du soul	Step 4 p. 23 Stress M, M/m, m, m/m	Step 5 p. 24 Ident. b, m, s, b/m/s	Step 6 p. 26 Manifestation	Step 7 p. 27 Who is involved?	Step 8 p. 29 Time	Step 9 p. 30 Origin	Step 10 p. 31 Clues	Step 11 p. 34 Emotional Gauge for HHH Dowsing Negative pp. 57, 58	Positive pp. 57, 63	Step 12 pp. 36, 105-114 Resolution	Step 13 p. 37 Always balance 100%
E	sb	M (Major)	M (Mind)	Central Nervous System	Friend Not my issue	About 2 monhs ago	My yard		Frustrated	Need to provide an ear	This is not my issue. I let go of the frustrated Energy which is held on my Subconscious level of my Being manifesting in my Central Nervous System. This energy no longer serves me. I provide an ear to listen to my friend Maxine. Thank You. Bless Love, Bless Love, Bless Love.	100%

for Step 3: c=conscious, sb=subconscious, sp=super-conscious, unc=unconscious, du=DUPI, soul=soul, ch=chosen, nc=not chosen

for Step 4: How much stress is involved: M=Major issue, M/m=Major/Minor issue, m=Minor issue, m/m=Minor/Minor issue

for step 5: b=body, m=mind, s=spirit, b/m/s=body and mind and spirit, o/u=Other or Unknown at this time

Emotional Gauge for HHH Dowsing

These energies or emotions can be created by yourself or by others. Find the most important positive energy and negative energy on this page for an issue. Also see additional *Negative Words* p. 58, additional *Positive Words* p. 63, and *Chakras* p. 73.

Positive Energy	Chakra Relates to Color and Attitude	Negative Energy
Determination Expect Hugging Onward Provide Seeking Truth and wholeness Wish	**Neo Brain** (above the Crown chakra) Transparent Clearing 8	Cast out Framed Inferior Irritated Lazy (Too) outspoken Speak out/up
Absolute Assurance At-one-ment Bliss Brand new Correct Encouraged Erect Expecting Involved Perfect	**Crown** White Appreciation 7	Behind Confused Encircled Fuming Loses Not listened to Pointed Pride Ruined Surprised Tight Youngster (immaturity)
Aware Buoyancy Comparable Determination Erect In tune Pride Relief	**Brow** Indigo Admiration 6	Encumbered Faded Left out Mean Resolved Tight Troubled Unselfish Vulgar Youngster (immaturity)
Abstain Assurance Beautiful Best Change Enjoy Fulfilled Involved Moving Precious Sign Simple Speak out/up (Too) outspoken Turn	**Throat** Blue Willing 5	Bold Challenged Directed Evoked Forgetting Hustled Intrenched Loveless Morbid Not generous Oppressed Outspoken Tempted Transgressed
Abstain Accommodate Attainment Buoyancy Clearing Compassion Compassionate Determination Divine Expect Loving Moving Perfect Precise Support Writing Youngster (immaturity)	**Heart** Green Attunement 4	Abject Embarrassed Emptiness Grumbling Hitched Introverted Morbid Persecuted Possessed Queer Rigid Rotted Stinky Yanking Youngster (immaturity)
Accomplish Adjusted Attuned Changeable Channel Coexist Decision Employ Enchantment Engaging Erect In tune Loving place Slender Turn	**Solar Plexus** Yellow Assurance 3	Antagonism Bribed Confused Defeated Depressed Evoked Frightened Frustrated Paralyzed
Acceptance Acquit Attuned Clearing Climbing Collected Delightful Elated Enfold Frugal Godly Knowing myself In time Precious Surprise Transition Wonder	**Sex** Orange Interest 2	Conquered Depressed Entangled Frightened Fuming Indifferent Loaded down Overreact Reform Seeking Void Zoned
Changeable Choosing Dynamic Employ Encouragement Enfold Godly Knowing Lord Peace Place Stability Trust	**Root** Red Oneness 1	Bereaved Conceited Humiliated Lied about or lied to Overcharged Oversensitive Rejected Sorry for self Trapped Troubled